AUSTRALIA'S NEW

AUSTRALIA'S NEW AGED

Issues for young and old

John McCallum & Karin Geiselhart

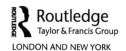
Routledge
Taylor & Francis Group

LONDON AND NEW YORK

To our parents and our children

First published 1996 by Allen & Unwin

Published 2020 by Routledge
2 Park Square, Milton Park, Abingdon, Oxon OX14 4RN
605 Third Avenue, New York, NY 10017

Routledge is an imprint of the Taylor & Francis Group, an informa business

National Library of Australia
Cataloguing-in-Publication entry:

McCallum, John, 1949 Oct. 3– .
    Australia's new aged: issues for young and old.

    Bibliography.
    Includes index.
    ISBN 1 86448 218 4.

    1. Aged—Government policy—Australia. 2. Aged—Care—Australia. 3. Aged—Home care—Australia. 4. Aged—Services for—Australia. 5. Aged—Health and hygiene—Australia. I. Geiselhart, Karin. II. Title.

362.60994

Set in 10.5/12pt Times by DOCUPRO, Sydney

ISBN-13: 9781864482188 (pbk)

Contents

Acknowledgments

I am grateful to Barbara Davison, Hal Kendig, Deirdre Jones, Victor Minichiello and David Walker for their comments on an earlier draft of this material.

I wish to also thank the Bondi Surf Bathers' Life Saving Club for permission to reproduce the artwork on p.19, and the University of Queensland Press for permission to reproduce Steele Rudd's 'Jim Takes A Hand', originally published in *Grandpa's Selection and Other Stories*, Angus and Robertson 1919, and now in Steele Rudd's *On Our Selection*, University of Queensland Press, 1984.

Introduction

The notion that our society is ageing has become a popular source of gloomy predictions for the future. We are warned that disproportionate numbers of feeble, dependent elders will place an unsupportable drain on our social welfare and health care systems. We have an image of today's youth struggling, in their mature years, to pay for the masses of geriatric baby boomers whose productive years lie far behind.

Like many widely accepted beliefs, this one is part reality, part myth. It is certain that the proportion of the population over 60, and particularly over 80, will steadily increase over the next four decades. Australia is no different from most developed countries in this respect. Indeed, some countries, including Sweden or more recently Japan, have experienced a far more rapid shift towards an older society, without a noticeable collapse in their social structure or economy.

It is easy to lose sight of the fact that the increase in the proportion of aged people, like many demographic movements, is itself a temporary phenomenon. By 2040 Australia's population will be more evenly distributed among the various age groups. Total numbers of each, however, will continue to expand, creating new variables for planners to consider. The challenge is to distinguish between solid trends and pure speculation, and develop policies which are flexible enough to adapt to new directions.

Like many social shifts, the ageing of our population is part of wider changes which may have unpredictable impacts. In the 1930s, who would have predicted the dramatic transformation of women's roles which has affected so many aspects of daily life? And who really knows now what the technologies of the 90s and beyond may mean for our work and play in future? Even climate change could have repercussions, presently unclear apart from some discussion of the medical implications.

Both public and private responses to social changes are usually slower and more recalcitrant than desirable. The widespread introduction of child care and computers, to give examples from the domestic and technological fields, brought with them conflict and confusion. Yet over a period of less than 20 years, they have become firmly established in our lives.

All we can be sure of is change. It is a safe bet that the retirement lives of tomorrow's elderly will differ at least as much from those of their parents as their working lives do now. Policies set for one cohort of elderly will not necessarily meet the needs or consumer tastes of new groups entering old age. Thinking has changed, for example, about the meaning and content of individual rights and citizenship.

The baby boom age cohort, now at its productive peak, will be retiring in droves 5 to 10 years after the turn of the century. As one of the healthiest and best educated, housed, and informed groups ever, they are likely to redefine retirement. They will be able to do this because, more than ever before, this group will be 'cashed-up' on superannuation and other investments, and this will give them unprecedented power. A disproportionate number of them will be women, many of whom broke new ground for their gender as breadwinners, activists, and consumers. This gives a different and potentially exciting perspective to the ageing of the population. National groups like the Older Women's Network are already seizing every opportunity to interact with the planners and program deliverers to make their needs known. This raises the interesting question: Where are the men? Early rumblings indicate that they may be moving to assert their own needs and views about ageing.

In every area from health care to housing to retirement income, the aged will be seeking to put their own views. They will not want to be sitting on the sidelines. But not all of tomorrow's aged will be active and affluent. Some will be poor, or disempowered because of their race or ethnic background. Growing inequalities affect incomes and opportunities. Thus older people's needs and resources in retirement will be as diverse as previously. The problem is that official reactions to this new phenomenon are not very thoughtful or sensitive.

The problem with the 'social problem' approach to ageing

Academics, policy-makers and activists alike have become trapped in a 'social problem' approach to ageing. Whatever the theme—nursing homes, abuse of the elderly, low rates of sexual intercourse, rising health costs—their strategy has been to declare that a crisis is imminent or already here and that someone will have to step in, usually government, to help the poor defenceless elderly. Such a claim can normally get a run in the media, and if it is really sensational, a front page with blanket media coverage for a day. Over the last 15 years we have assumed that the elderly area homogeneous, disadvantaged group with common interests. We have had to stop them 'double dipping' into the pension system, but protect them from rapacious and callous nursing home operators, stop them from bankrupting the health system, but 'allow' them to live at home as long as possible, and so on. All these are things that have been done for them as 'a defenceless and disadvantaged group' without much serious participation from their representative groups. Many of these policy changes were directed by people with little or no contact with elderly people in the settings for which policy was being formulated.

It is not hard to see the weakness with our social problem strategy for dealing with ageing. The elderly are not universally disadvantaged and defenceless. Many are well off and most exercise power in family and social groups. They are increasingly unhappy with being talked about as though they were unable to decide for themselves and having things done for them rather than with and by them. Instead of grabbing headlines with misleading horror stories and adopting a defender role for the elderly, academics, activists and policy-makers are going to have to become more professional, to exchange their social problem approach for a social scientific one that considers evidence on the public record and genuinely engages the elderly in the process of policy-making. This requires a major shift in the reporting of ageing issues by the media.

The following story is at least one trend in American popular reporting that we could hope to see emulated in Australia! It is curious that negative American stories, like those about 'granny dumping', are widely reported in Australia while positive stories are not picked up by our media at all.

Like your grandfather's Oldsmobile, the image of an America debilitated by age belongs to a different economy and an earlier generation. Instead, a series of broad, mutually reinforcing changes in the US economy will make an aging population much more of an economic asset than before . . .

Companies now use information technologies to raise productivity. And higher productivity . . . makes it easier to fund the Social Security and health care bills that are squeezing American's wallet today.

Another change is that people can be more productive far longer in an information-and-services economy than one dominated by factories and heavy industry. Healthier lifestyles and medical advances should also postpone disability among the elderly.

Business Week, 12/9/94, cover story.

The book

This book sets out the predictable parameters that will affect planning for this increase in older people over the middle term, namely to the year 2020—that is, when most of the readers of this book (and certainly the authors) will themselves be moving into a different life stage.

We cannot promise you a totally dispassionate look at the major issues for an ageing Australia. However, we hope to give at least a clear outline of them, and to distinguish, wherever possible, between the facts and the illusions. We have attempted to bring together a wide range of relevant research and published statistics while keeping our focus on desirable outcomes.

At every point, critical questions are raised: What is the true purpose of this policy or program? Who is really benefiting, and how does this fit into an agenda of achieving the greatest social good? Policies, programs and social constructs for the aged are, like all others, part of the whirl of the political, economic and bureaucratic 'marketplace'. Outcomes emerge, sometimes as a result of chaotic processes whose end result is unpredictable and very dependent on the initial assumptions. True rationalism doesn't always prevail. Hence the strong emphasis in the following chapters on empowerment, accountability, and information sharing.

We have written this book for students of the social sciences, policy-makers, those who set up programs in the community and others who want to be informed about and influence future directions of care and planning for the aged. The opportunity for action is now, not the next century when the baby boom generations retire and grow old. We intend this book to contribute to the development of a cohesive yet flexible approach to ageing policy.

1

Our ageing population: Part of a global wave

Concerned reporting of the ageing of Australia is not a recent development. It has become a regular topic of media attention. For example, some 20 years ago Dr William McBride pronounced his views on population ageing in the *Women's Weekly* in 1976.[1]

> How can a declining and progressively ageing population, which isn't even replacing itself, sustain a modern country? Remember, too, that where a population is ageing, greater burdens fall on the diminishing pool of the young . . . The ramifications are endless. The whole structure of life must change.

At the time, McBride was at the peak of his career. For his discovery that thalidomide causes birth defects, McBride was awarded a CBE (Commander of the British Empire) in 1969 and the French L'Institut de la Vie in 1971, and was named Australian Father of the Year in 1972. Sensationally, he was struck off the NSW Medical Register in 1993 for falsifying scientific evidence in another investigation. We may well question whether his dire warnings about an ageing society were based on fact.

A lot has happened since McBride made those statements, not least a chronic unemployment problem in the developed world. Similar concerns in Australia, along with worries about our 'carrying capacity' as a continent, have contributed to a drop in immigration levels, following some intense debate. And amid global recognition that there are simply too many people of all ages everywhere, the comparatively modest increases projected for Australia's aged take on a less urgent cast.

But some ideas are just too convenient to fade away. Some respected authorities are still calling on women to produce more babies to counter the growing burden of an ageing society. Fertility is still perceived by some as the cargo cult pathway to preserving a way of life endangered by unproductive old people.

This chapter questions the legitimacy of such forecasts about an ageing Australia. Does the evidence support this grim picture? It fits nicely with another popular belief, that people roughly over 50 are 'past it', in a steady downward decline of their mental and physical prowess. The metaphors 'over the hill' and 'no spring chicken' sum up a comfortable but negative generalisation of ageing. Is a decreasing pool of young people doomed to support growing legions of greying and decaying elders? Demographics, the science of vital and social statistics, can help answer these questions.

The numbers alone can never give the full picture. We need to examine the demographics together with their context, the larger waves of human trends and changing social conditions. Today's 'oldies' are not just growing in numbers—they are also increasing their share of wealth and political influence. Unprecedented social changes since World War II in family size, gender roles, ethnic composition, employment mobility, education levels and life-style expectations have made the coming crop of middle aged more demanding and powerful than ever before. Yet our social institutions are still largely geared to 'Gran' back in 'Blue Hills' days. Rather than 'over the hill', it may be more appropriate to speak of older people 'storming the hill', 'taking the high ground' and holding onto it.

The critical problem arising from population ageing is not one of excessive burdens imposed on the young, as McBride had claimed, but the slowness of social and economic institutions to accommodate an unprecedented range of fundamental changes in our society, like the medium-term rise in the numbers of elderly. It is extremely unlikely, on current trends, that higher birth rates or immigration levels will reverse this ageing of the population. McBride was partly right when he said the structure of society will have to change. But we argue that it is the social and economic structures rather than the demography that has to change.

Where these changes should occur and how they can most fully meet the needs of an increasing proportion of elderly is the subject of the rest of this book. We support policies that are based on broadly acquired evidence. Decision-makers should make this evidence accessible to interested groups and, through the media, to the general public. Only then can they formulate and voice their views confidently. In this chapter the basic population trends underlying the ageing of Australian society are presented. The next chapter puts these in their social, policy and economic context. Together these form the background for the subsequent chapters in which major issues such as retirement income, health and community services are analysed.

Population ageing—how much and how fast?

Demographers define aged populations as those with 10 per cent or more at 65+ years, or with 15 per cent or more at 60+ years. By these definitions, Australia had a mature population in 1971 and an aged population in 1991. This increase in the proportions of older groups was wrought by changes in three underlying forces: birth, death and immigration rates.

There is much to be learned from the representation of Australia's age groups by the so-called population pyramid, which shows the distribution of a population's age groups by gender (see Figure 1.1). The shape of the pyramid changes according to birth, death and immigration rates. If a population had an equal number of males and females at every age, the pyramid would be fully symmetrical. Because females outlive males, the pyramid becomes skewed towards females at the top. In theory, mature and ageing populations, such as Australia, could eventually look like inverted pyramids, with larger proportions of older groups, and relatively small proportions in younger groups. A totally stable population would look more like a pillar, with nearly equal proportions moving through each age group. For the purposes of our analysis in this chapter, the proportions of age groups, or cohorts, in their productive years (roughly 15–64) are the ones to watch because the size of these groups relative to the combined top and bottom groups is what tells us whether the aged will dominate in numbers.[2]

In the 1971 Census, population proportions approximate a pyramid, with only two periods creating unevenness in the slope. These 'blips' embody history, past and future respectively. Between ages 30 to 39 there is an indent in the side of the pyramid indicating lower birth rates for those age cohorts. This phenomenon occurred during the 1930s when the Great Depression led to lower birth rates and fewer marriages. Then at the base, from ages 0 to 10 years, the lower proportions of children characteristic of the change to an ageing population are already in evidence. The bulk of the population is of working age, with large numbers of dependent children and relatively few aged.

Figure 1.1 Population pyramids for 1971, 1991, 2011, 2031

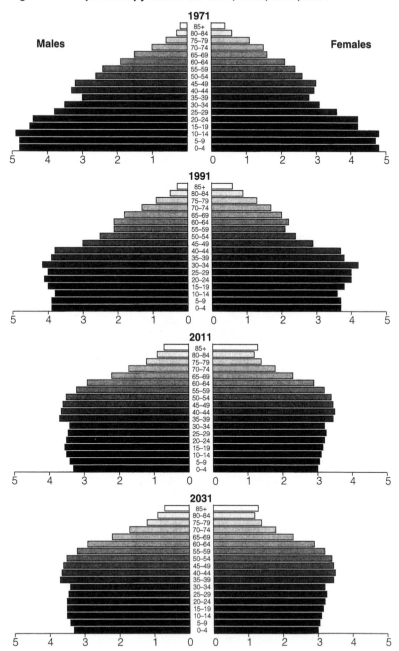

In the 1991 Census data the shape is changing from a pyramid to a bell. Again the base of the bell is characterised by relatively small and relatively equal proportions in the ages 0 to 14 years. The baby boom age cohorts can be seen bulging out above the younger groups. There is a benefit from this as the small Australian Depression birth cohorts are now reaching retirement ages. We are in the 'golden years' for managing an ageing population, with the baby boomers in the workforce and relatively small groups of both young and old. However, they will be 'golden years' only if we use them to save for the future and establish prudent public policies.

The projections for 2011 are now the shape of a bell with smaller proportions at younger ages. As the baby boomers enter retirement ages, the 'golden years' end and the peak years of the ageing population begin. It shows us clearly the growth of the 'old' old, 80+ years, which began almost imperceptibly in the 1970s. In fact, the Australian Bureau of Statistics consistently under-predicted the numbers of very old Australians who would be alive during the 1970s. This was because older Australians started to live even longer as diseases like coronary heart disease had less impact. So we see 'ageing at the top' of the pyramid, and the age groups increasing most rapidly are the 'old' old. Yet even in 2011 the proportion of the population of working age does not fall below 1961 levels.

The 2031 projections show the population becoming more like a barrel with relatively smooth sides due to equal proportions in most age groups. This should remind us that, in the longer term, a rapidly ageing population is a temporary phenomenon. Some time around the middle of the next century the relative imbalances between age groups will have worked through, most people will survive from birth to advanced old age and the population will reach a new stable state. Only around this time do the proportions of working versus dependent fall below 1981 levels.

The years 2030 and beyond will be the adult years for today's teenagers and children. They will depend on us to get the policy mix right for an ageing population but also to establish structures suitable for a stable population 40 years from now.

The immigration option

It is often suggested that higher levels of immigration would help to offset the effects of an ageing population. However, this is politically unlikely and probably environmentally unsound. Professor Lincoln Day, previously of the Australian National University, estimates that continued immigration at 1988 levels will result in an extra 7 million people by the year 2022, whereas with no immigration, population would stabilise at around 20 million by then—that is, at about 2 million more. It has been argued for some time that immigration only postpones the problem, as immigrants also grow old and become dependent. It may also be true that an aged population is less demanding on resources in some respects: housing construction, education and child care.

> Older age structures, as such, need not substantially elevate the demands on a country's resources . . . We see no insurmountable obstacles to preventing urban-industrial countries from developing acceptable programs that would simultaneously enable more people to be employed, achieve substantial savings, and create healthier environments. Whether such programs are actually undertaken is another matter. But it is a matter not of money or age structure; it is a matter of social priorities and power relations between different sectors of the society.[3]
>
> A.T. Day and L.H. Day, *'The Lay of the Land'. Old Age Structures, Environment and Social Change.*

Drawing concepts of biological sustainability, Dr Timothy Flannery[4] of the Australian Museum maintains that we have already passed our optimum population level, as we have degraded 70 per cent of the cropping soils. He puts our ideal population at the lower end of 6 to 12 million. Note that such estimates of 'carrying capacity' are based on the optimistic assumption that conditions will not deteriorate appreciably. Thus, although Dr Flannery reminds us that Australia is a land of extremes and unpredictable weather, neither he nor anyone else can yet say with certainty whether global climactic change will in fact eventuate, or with what impact on this continent. Bearing in mind that the global reinsurance industry, which covers the risk of insurers, is now worried about such possibilities, a conservative approach to population growth may well be warranted. These new ideas may influence the future shape of our ageing population in ways that are as yet unknown.

The growth of the 'old' old

As well as discussing an overall picture of the age groups, it is important to look at relative changes within the aged population itself. Between 1971 and 2031 the absolute numbers of people aged 85 years and over is expected to increase by a factor of 10. The population proportions of women aged 85+ increase from half a per cent in 1971 to almost three per cent in 2031. By contrast, the proportions of the population aged 0 to 14 years decline from 22 per cent in 1991 to 17 per cent in 2031. The numbers of those aged 65+ will treble between 1991 and 2031, 1.9 million to 5.2 million. The obvious imbalance in the sexes that is evident in the pyramids becomes even more pronounced at older ages. The 'old' old groups are predominantly female with only 52 men per 100 women aged 85+ expected in 2031. Clearly we must accept that living to an advanced age has become a normal experience. It remains for us to understand the full implications and to adjust our social institutions to deal with the changes.

In summary, what does the population 'pyramid' analysis tell us? Through the 1990s and early years of the next century Australia has large population proportions of workforce age and small groups of young and old. Around 2011 Australia's peak birth and immigration rates of post-World War II years which produced its baby boom begins to affect the sizes of groups at retirement ages. By 2031 the baby boomers enter the 'old' old group aged 80 years and above.

The ageing of the baby boomers to the year 2011 will create needs for pensions, housing and leisure facilities. The movement of the baby boom into 'old' old ages will create a need for aged care facilities like nursing homes and community services to support older people at home.

Australia—a youthful country amid ageing neighbours?

Australia's post-World War II baby boom was boosted by unprecedented levels of young adult immigrants. This amplified the effects of already high birth rates. However, as the pyramid shows, the word 'boom' implies too much 'bang' for the Australian case! The so-called baby boom would be better described as a baby 'plateau' encompassing ages 15 to 44 in 1991. By contrast the baby booms of Canada and USA cover a narrower age span of about 25 to 44 years and in Japan it was even more narrow. These countries have much lower levels of immigration. Japan, for example, has almost none and neither the benefits nor costs of multiculturalism.

As a consequence of this long period of high population growth Australia is not experiencing acute population ageing by world standards—it has one of the youngest populations of any developed Western nation. European countries like Sweden already have proportions of populations aged 60+ above 20 per cent and continue to operate generous welfare states with no more crisis in their economies than other countries have. In countries like Sweden 1 out of every 5 people you are likely to meet will be elderly. By contrast, Australia in 1995 had 1 in 8 (about 12 per cent aged 60+).

Nor is the Australian speed of ageing particularly notable. It is estimated that it will take Great Britain 86 years to move from 10 to 20 per cent of its population aged 60+. The projections for Sweden and Australia are 68 years and 45 years respectively.[5] By comparison, Japan is expected to take 22 years and ageing will have accelerated to occur by 2006. Similarly rapid ageing is occurring in Hong Kong, Singapore and the other fast-developing countries of the Asia Pacific region. So Australia's population is ageing moderately and doing so in the most rapidly ageing region of the world.

The ethnic mosaic

Given this regional disparity in rates of ageing, it is perhaps surprising that immigrants are the most rapidly ageing group in the Australian population. While the Australian-born 60+ population is expected to increase by 25 per cent between 1981 and 2001, the corresponding increase for the overseas-born is 110 per cent. The elderly from non-English-speaking countries will comprise a majority of the overseas-born elderly by 2001 with increases of something like 350 per cent for groups such as those from Greece. Healthier people find their way to the front of migration queues over those who are less healthy. The healthy migrant effect evident in longer lives is especially pronounced for Greeks and Italians. These differences are large enough that we should consider the ethnic aged, in some respects, separately from the general population. The ultimate objective must be to truly recognise the multicultural nature of ageing in Australia.

Various ethnic groups in the first generation have different proportions of elderly (See Figure 1.2). In the 1991 Census only 6 per cent of Vietnamese were 60+ compared to 9 per cent of Lebanese and 34 per cent of Italians. Migrants from Italy and the Netherlands came in relatively high numbers during the 1950s and then numbers from these sources reduced to a mere trickle. Consequently 8 per cent of those

**Figure 1.2   Proportions of people aged 50+ years from various
birthplace groups, 1991**

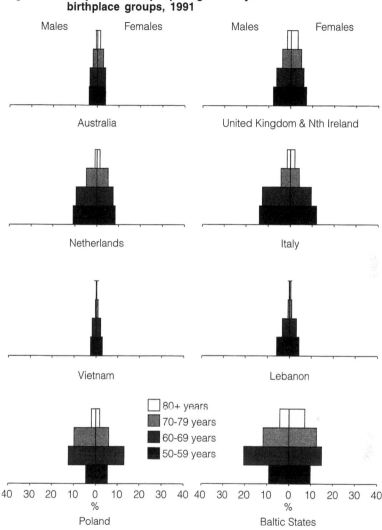

Source: Australian Bureau of Statistics, 1991 Census

born in Italy and 10 per cent of those from the Netherlands were aged
70–79 in 1986 compared to 5 per cent of Australian-born. The proportions of those aged 70–79 years from Poland and the Baltic States
(Estonia, Latvia and Lithuania) are extreme at 16 per cent and 24 per
cent respectively. In addition there are atypical sex ratios for Poles,

with 192 males per 100 females aged 80–89 in 1991 compared to 71 for Australian-born. Not only did they arrive in considerable numbers in the late 1940s and then almost cease for 25 years, but disproportionate numbers of them were men, many of whom remained unmarried. By contrast, Vietnamese who arrived mostly during the late 1970s and 1980s have only one per cent aged 70–79.

These factors are important for understanding the diversity of need among aged Australians. First, about a quarter of Australians aged 50–70 do not speak English well and for those aged 75+ this increases to a third. Second, there are cultural preferences, for example for food, among migrant groups. Australia's elderly population is not only growing but in the process becoming more ethnically diverse. Those from non-English-speaking backgrounds, and immigrants generally, will contribute disproportionately to the ageing of the Australian population. As with the non-migrant population, women will be increasingly over-represented as this group ages.

From the broader picture we can identify three stages in the ageing of immigrant populations. First there is the ageing of the working-age immigrant group who begin to enter retirement usually in a healthy state. This has already occurred for the early groups of post-World War II migrants. Second, the increasing concentrations of 'old' old immigrants create demands for culturally appropriate community services. We expect this process now for Baltic States and later for other groups. Third, there is the ageing of the Australian-born children of immigrants through similar stages to 1 and 2. Little is known about how ethnic origins will affect circumstances and needs in the second generation. In 1991 half of Australian-born people with one or more parents born overseas were less than 30 years old, and the proportions of those 60+ were around 1 per cent. An exception were those of German descent, with more than 15 per cent aged 60+. The growth of the aged in the second generation of immigrants will be largely an issue for the next century with more urgent present concerns about the ageing of the first generation in immigrant groups.

Our indigenous old

Minority groups cannot be examined in the general population analysis since their experiences are lost in the averages dominated by majority groups. Aborigines and Torres Strait Islanders (ATSI) have not enjoyed the increased longevity of the rest of the Australian population. In the 1991 Census only 4 per cent of the indigenous population was aged

Figure 1.3 Distribution of older people, Aborigines and Torres Strait Islanders and the non-Aboriginal population, 1991

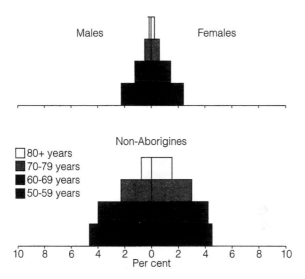

Source: Australian Bureau of Statistics, 1991 Census

60+ compared to 16 per cent of the non-indigenous. The most striking feature is the high death rate of young and middle-aged adult Aborigines. While the death rates of Aborigines are comparable with those in less developed countries, the causes of death are quite different. The infectious diseases that are so destructive in developing countries are less prevalent; ischaemic heart disease and stroke are the leading killers. For older indigenous people the death rates actually approximate those for the rest of the population, the damage having been done at younger ages. This sobering story, a national disgrace, is lost in the aggregated population figures for all Australia. It is a scandal requiring a complete national response in its own right, and not as a small addendum to reforms to policies on ageing.

The bottom line—cost projections

The heavy media pressure promoting doomsday visions of an ageing society has motivated several comprehensive studies of the costs of an ageing population. It did not take long to convert population numbers into dollars. Generally speaking the cost projections do not add up to expenditure growth of crisis proportions.

The first Commonwealth Economic Planning Advisory Council (EPAC) analysis published in 1988[6] made very moderate assessments of costs to the year 2025. It presented evidence that expenditures on social security and welfare, education and employment would rise by an average 1.3 per cent a year. Welfare and health expenditures would increase over the period but would be offset by declining education outlays. Maintaining the levels of per capita expenditure with an ageing population could be covered by a 0.3 per cent annual increase in labour productivity. If the share of social expenditures were to increase in line with productivity growth to maintain the relative income of older people, the costs would be greater. The authors of the EPAC analysis correctly point to the uncertainties of projections over 40 years and several of their suggestions, including options on superannuation, have influenced policies subsequently.

The second analysis, published 6 years later in 1994,[7] carried out ambitious projections to the year 2051. It expected welfare expenditures (not including pensions) on people 65+ to remain stable at about 3.4 per cent of gross domestic product (GDP). Including pensions, these expenditures were expected to rise from 6.9 per cent of GDP in 1990 to 7.9 per cent in 2051. This very modest rise reflects the impacts of the superannuation policy changes which are discussed at length in Chapter 3. Without these reforms the proportion of GDP would be 9.3 per cent of GDP in 2051 as against 7.9 per cent with them.

The report is most concerned about rising health care expenditures in an ageing population. It projects an increase in aggregate health care expenditures from $29 billion in 1990 to $126 billion in 2051, a rise from 8.4 per cent to 11.1 per cent of GDP which is attributable to an ageing population. While currently about one third of health expenditures go to people aged 65+ this could increase to more than 50 per cent by 2051, according to the report. As discussed in Chapter 4, the methods used to project costs are not in accord with recent evidence. Studies of actual health cost increases show that ageing is a very minor part of the process in Australia and internationally.

From the same population projections we can expect nursing home, hostels and Home and Community Care costs to increase from $2 to $7 billion between 1991 and 2051. Relative to health cost projections, the aged care service costs were only 7.9 per cent of health costs in 1991 and decline to 5.8 per cent in 2051.

The report correctly notes that ageing implications cannot be limited to analyses for the 65+ population. It has implications for schools, universities, the greying of the workforce, and the structure and demands on families. Both EPAC reports also consider how immigration can moderate the costs of ageing. The most recent report takes this debate further by placing it in the context of ecologically sustainable development, not just in the context of economic and population growth.

We do need to be cautious with any projections that take us 60 years into the future. By 2051 we expect that the Australian population will no longer be an ageing one but will have reached a stable state with lower birth rates. Even if these projections are accurate, they do not represent an imminent crisis. There is a demand for reasonable policies and cost management but short-term, kneejerk reactions are unwarranted.

Conclusion

We can summarise the population trends revealed in demographic analysis as follows:

1 increasing proportions of the population in retirement ages but not dramatically so until the first decade of the next century;
2 rapidly increasing numbers of 'old' old (80+) occurring through the 1990s;
3 feminisation of the elderly, especially the 'old' old;
4 extreme ageing in some first-generation migrant groups; and
5 a failure of the ATSI populations to reach old age.

These changes are occurring in the context of a growing economy and a dynamic society. They are now cloaked with a rhetoric of crisis in headlines such as 'tidal waves' of the aged swamping a diminishing pool of the young. Our analysis shows that due to these demographic changes several sectors of need are growing, but only to a moderate extent compared to other developed countries. The Australian evidence for this consistently indicates that ageing does not present an economic crisis. The trend is clearly manageable within the constraints of a modest growth rate according to all reports, most recently the national Economic Planning and Advisory Council.

Alarmist headline writers project demographic figures and pretend nothing else will change or adapt. We can expect that compensating social and economic changes will alter the impact of demographic change. Thus demographic forces must be analysed in a social and political context. Even considering the demography alone, there are proportionally only as many dependent children and elderly today as there were in the 1960s. Hence we challenge the extravagant claims of writers like Dr McBride with a rhetorical question: Crisis—what crisis?

Notes

1 McBride, Dr William, 'The Vanishing Australian', *The Australian Women's Weekly*, 25 August 1976, p. 16–17.
2 Demographic data used in Chapter 1 are derived from Australian Bureau of Statistics Censuses and Population Projections.
3 Day, A. T. & Day, L. H., 1994, *'The Lay of the Land'. Old Age Structures, Environment and Social Change: Opportunities for Australia and the Netherlands in the 21st Century*, The Netherlands Interdisciplinary Demographic Institute, Amsterdam, p. 16
4 Flannery, T., 1991, 'Australia: overpopulated or last frontier?', *Australian Natural History*, 23 (10).
5 McCallum, J., 1995, 'Exporting aged care services to Asia: Regional trends and Australian responses'. In J. McCallum (ed.) *Export of Aged Care Services Training*, National Centre for Epidemiology and Population Health, Canberra.
6 Economic Planning and Advisory Council 1988, *Economic Effects of an Ageing Population*, EPAC, Canberra.
7 Economic Planning and Advisory Council 1994, *Australia's Ageing Society*, EPAC, Canberra.

2

Post-modern ageing: Unpicking poorly knit structures

The demographic forces that define population ageing are commonly represented by the metaphor of a tidal wave with destructive consequences for social and economic life. Metaphors that capture the public imagination have the potential to drive public opinion and policy reforms and, therefore, must be taken seriously. However, the evidence in this book shows that the flow-through from demographic change to social and economic costs is, at best, indirect, if it exists at all. Progress can be achieved by improving the metaphors that influence policy so that our interventions can be more effective.

Social consequences of ageing are not predetermined by demography. They are the product of historic policies and public attitudes which are changeable or at least modifiable. In this sense the consequences of ageing are 'socially constructed'. They are produced by social attitudes and by people deliberately following or blindly conforming to social norms. Even the metaphors for ageing like the 'tidal wave' are themselves constructed by powerful opinion leaders using their influence over the media! They are either trying to make it a 'good' story or even to create pressure for public sector cost cutting which may be of benefit to them.

Nursing home expenditures grew logarithmically in the 1970s, a time when the population of Australians 70 years and over was low and stable. It was simply considered a good thing to provide 'homes' for older people and the policy was a political boon to the Menzies government when it was introduced in the 1960s. The 'ageist' attitude, which allows people to derive satisfaction from doing things for older people who are presumed

15

to be useless and dependent, has deep historical roots in Australia. The fact that older people themselves largely detested and feared 'old people's homes' was lost in the enthusiasm of politicians for opening new buildings. The dramatic increase in nursing home costs was not driven by the demography of ageing, nor by the wishes of the aged, but by 'ageist' values and political self-interest.

We need to be actively critical of claims about population ageing if we are to deal with the political and social issues it raises. Various critical methods are now used by academics. One of these, 'deconstruction', is an appropriate method to deal with claims involving demographic determinism. Like lawyers fighting the case for older people we need to challenge both the quality of evidence being presented and the credibility and integrity of those making the claims.[1] A 'critical realist' sense of deconstruction is advocated for discussing ageing. Unlike the application of deconstruction to literary texts, where truth and outcomes are fluid, it does matter for policy-making what the evidence is and where the truth lies. We are encouraging everyone involved to challenge more vigorously the claims and conventions about ageing and to make a more critical use of the wide-ranging evidence about the claims. Only by criticising the claims—for example that increasing numbers of older people per se require policy changes—can we make progress with changing policies and social attitudes in ways that allow full citizenship to older people.

Current generations of older people are taking on the task of challenging social policies and attitudes with the support of oncoming cohorts of middle-aged baby boomers. Rather than evoking a destructive tidal wave, we should choose a new set of attitudes, values and expectations to define older people. Like a poorly made sweater, the social structures limiting older people have to be unpicked and re-knitted. To succeed in this task we need to grasp the character of contemporary Australian society.

A post-modern perspective on population ageing

Population ageing is quintessentially a 'post-modern' phenomenon, to use the current theoretical language. It is an outcome of successful modernisation and a characteristic feature of post-modern societies. 'Post-modernism' and 'deconstructionism' are theories coined by social thinkers to deal with the complexity and loss of singular certainty about truth and right in contemporary societies.[2] Post-modernists draw attention to the problem that the foundations of modern cultures in ideas of rationality, freedom, individualism and continual progress have been achieved at the expense of silenced minorities. 'Certainty' in social views was achieved by the exclusion of minority viewpoints. Claims of discrimination or oppression against women, the aged or indigenous Australians were seldom taken seriously. Recovery of their minority view is critical to the development of citizenship for the elderly and in that sense the deconstruction agenda is an appealing one for our task.

We need to be wary, however, of glib generalisations that derive from 'big' theories such as post-modernism. As one example, the problems of ageing existed long before the industrialisation of agricultural societies and the appearance of 'dark and satanic mills'. There was no idyllic social state in which older people lived harmoniously with their families in caring village communities. British historical studies have shown that the elderly were not much better or worse off in the early 17th century than they were at the end of the 19th century—years spanning the industrialisation of Britain.[3] About the same proportions of older people lived in three-generation households at the two periods almost three centuries apart. The decisive change in attitudes towards older people came late in the era of industrialisation with the development of pensions and aged care services. Nor did these idyllic conditions occur in continental Europe or Asia where other Australians have origins and where historical processes were different.

It is necessary to focus on diverse histories of ageing in various countries and at different times if we are to grasp the true roots of current attitudes to older people. There is no single broad process of modernisation encompassing all countries. All history is predominantly local and theoretical generalisations are only helpful as starting points. The task for Australians in search of a national identity is to understand why older people do not have a significant place in it except as dependent individuals in need of benevolent care. Grasping this process will enable us to turn around values and attitudes that limit the participation of older people. This task has not been a high priority one among Australian social historians.

The Australian identity is optimistic, uncomplicated and youthful. The reasons for the obsession with youth are historical as well as contemporary. This identity emerged from a desire to contrast a youthful Australia with an aged England, the old country, and an optimistic society with the cynicism of established cultures. Australia was also creating a new society so the image of youth was seductive. In the past Australia has been symbolised by a young boy or a young, adult, male Bondi lifesaver. The images of the aged are far less flattering—stooped, crazy, useless and dependent.

Ageism may be the next frontier of Australian historiography. In spite of the burgeoning literature on Australian social history that has now embraced Aborigines, women, homosexuals, migrants and a host of other sub-groups, barely one serious article has been published in recent years on the history of old age . . . Compared with the United States, where no fewer than eight major studies of the history of old age have appeared since the late 1970s, or Britain, where a group of historians in Cambridge have revolutionised our understanding of the place of old people in pre-industrial society, older people are still largely missing from Australia's history books.[4]

Graeme Davison, *Old People in a Young Society: Towards a History of Ageing in Australia.*

The peculiar combination of forces at large during the period when nationhood was achieved may have made Australia one of the most ageist cultures in the developed world.[5] Because it was an immigrant society, it lacked grandparents. Very low proportions of Australians, 1 in 10 or even less, throughout our history have been reared with a grandparent under the same roof. For many, their grandparents remained in their country of origin or lived in another state. The complete separation from grandparents is still true of immigrant families today. The lack of relationships and ignorance about older people was accompanied by a benevolent attitude to their support. This desire to support the aged in Australia, but not through the degrading workhouse system of England, led to the early development of the aged pension. This benevolent paternalism helped older people but excluded them from the workforce. It created a group all with the same flat-rate income and with the derogatory label 'old age pensioners'. New images of the elderly have to be constructed and promoted to counteract these anachronistic images.

Culture and new technology

In this century Australian society has moved on at breakneck pace. Advanced forms of information technology and modern communications have transformed the fundamental character of work, leisure and

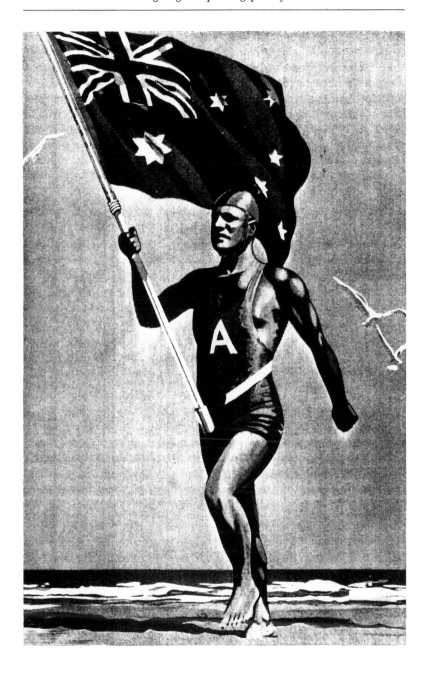

culture. Uniform values and consensual future visions no longer hold the imagination of the public. There are no longer any universally accepted manners or standards of behaviour. Some yearn for a more ecologically sustainable life, others for more conventional economic development based on immigration and population growth. No one view of the world enables the majority to pursue a single direction. The new media and information technologies of the 1990s alter people's access to knowledge and raise their expectations of material consumption and quality of services.

Along with swift technological change has come a revision of the rights of citizenship. The purchasing and voting power of consumers has become a force for the democratisation of public policies. Women have made great strides in claiming full citizenship, although many remain second-class citizens in economic terms. Claims for further reforms on the basis of gender sometimes lack perspective on class differences. There is mounting evidence that social inequalities based on income and location are increasing, and that they override and subsume those based on gender alone. But this perspective on an old and intractable problem is not politically popular.

Ageing and industrialisation

Population ageing is the product of successful industrialisation and a challenge to the social structures it established. The patterning of sex roles with men at work and women at home in nurturing and caring roles serviced the needs of industrial society. Similarly the male life-cycle pattern of education/training followed by work and independence and, finally, retirement and withdrawal from social roles, was fitted to the industrial work pattern. Few of these patterns remain, but the stereotypes persist. Older theories of ageing,[6] like disengagement theory which argued for voluntary social withdrawal in old age, or 'roleless' role theory which depicted old age as socially empty, reacted negatively to the contradictions of ageing in post-industrial society. Older people have generally presented happier and more positive images than these theories predicted.

The unilinear life-cycle is collapsing and the timing of life events, like parenthood and marriage, is becoming a matter of choice. Retirement is under challenge and age discrimination in employment has been outlawed in some states. The linear passage from work to old age was only ever true for men, not women. 'Post-modern' values only recently enshrined in legislation oppose the exclusion of women from work and

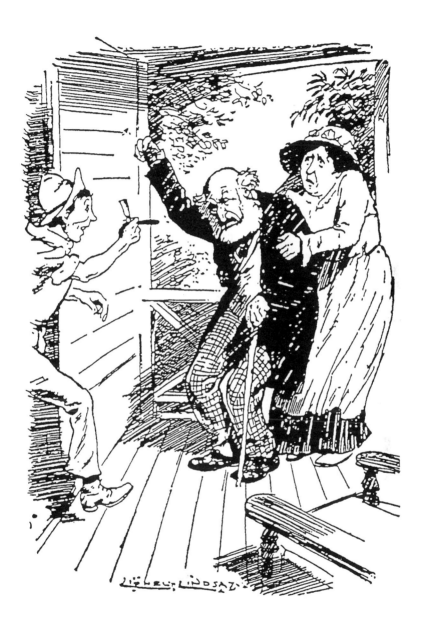

'There's no Poison, Grandpa,' Jim shouted,
'but Here's Your Razor'.

the forced withdrawal of older people at retirement ages. There are more women in the workforce and the roles of men and women in households are slowly changing.

Legislative structures are also moving slowly to allow a wider range of roles for the aged. Their institutionalisation in nursing homes for 'social' reasons has been challenged. A new process of assessing the suitability of people with health and care needs for reformed institutions has begun, and 'social admissions' have been de-institutionalised. Home and community care has been provided to enable frail older people to live decent lives as full citizens of the nation. Consultative processes are becoming the norm in public policy but are largely initiated and controlled by government bureaucracies.

The achievement of equal citizenship for the aged is not complete, in fact it has just begun. Citizenship requires the right of access to the social, economic and political life of the country and adequate means with which to exercise those rights. Current older people have rejected the popular, bio-medical assumptions that they are over the hill and are beginning to storm the hill to grasp their citizenship rights. We expect the claim to be carried forward even more strongly by new generations of people entering older age groups. A whole range of structural factors stand in their way, some obvious and some subtle but fundamental to Australian culture.

Structural shift[7]

The demographic shifts in numbers between age groups can be compared to movements of the plates of the earth's surface: they rub against one another, normally at imperceptible speed, but generate earthquakes and eruptions in some places. When the demographic forces confront rigid social structures political 'eruptions' are likely to occur. Ageing might just be the 'San Andreas fault' in the structure of modern Australian society!

In this clash demography is important but it is often only a minor part of the problem. If people ageing now would behave as their parents did, planning might be easier. But growing numbers of older people with money and satisfactory health are actively resisting stereotyped 'grey' roles in old age. They are slipping out of the ill-fitting, old-fashioned dresses into bicycle pants and runners. Their expectations of social involvement, regardless of their age and of the means and access to satisfy those expectations, are increasing. A core of radical activists are now elderly and organising others, more compliant in their earlier years, to voice their concerns as elderly Australians. They are seeking a 'grey' liberation in much the same way as women did in the 1970s. Indeed many of the elderly activists are women schooled in the protests of that era.

In response to structural shift, the Commonwealth and some state governments have undertaken thoroughgoing policy reviews. Consumer consultation has been a feature of such reviews. The rhetoric is excellent but the internal reforms for bureaucracies are more difficult than the policy statements. The inertia in government departments and the assumptions of staff that the elderly are over the hill present obstacles to achieving full citizenship for the aged. This recalcitrance parallels practices in business organisations, for example, which resist age discrimination in employment legislation.

The content of Australian citizenship has increased during this century. While legal rights to residency and voting provide the core of citizenship, these matter little without the material means to enjoy those rights. This understanding of a wider sense of Australian citizenship for older people was supported by the enactment of age pension legislation in 1908. In more recent years, there has been a move to protect these rights further with anti-discrimination legislation. People cannot enjoy their rights as Australian citizens if they suffer discrimination, which is sometimes an elusive phenomenon. It may be revealed only in resistance to legitimate demands or blindness to the obvious needs of older people.

Structural blindness and brutality

The social issues arising from demographic shifts are complex and easily subjected to untrue claims in the media and political debates. Resistance to changes, such as the growing numbers of older people, is a natural human instinct which can become insensitive and even vicious when it diminishes older people's quality of life. A case from the 1980s is that of Marie Anstee, who was retired by her employer at 60 even though 65 was the retiring age for male employees. In 1985 she successfully pursued her employer for sex discrimination before the NSW Anti-Discrimination Board. She argued that she had as much need of work income to pay off a mortgage as a man. The case was won on sex discrimination grounds rather than age which then was not recognised under the Act. Employers seldom act deliberately to hurt the interests of older workers. They are simply blind to their needs. This is typical of the problems of an ageing society: few of them are now related to demography.

Case 1: Marie Anstee v Allders International Pty Limited

Equal Opportunity Tribunal, No. 45 of 1984

On 6 February 1984, Ms Marie Anstee of Paddington, Sydney, complained to the President of the NSW Anti-Discrimination Board, alleging that she had been discriminated against on the ground of her sex in her employment by Allders International Pty Ltd. Ms Anstee was born in 1924 and she left her employment in 1984, after being terminated by her employer on reaching age 60.

In its 'decision on jurisdiction' of 10 July 1985 the Tribunal was unable to conclude that it had no jurisdiction in the case. It found that nothing in the 1982 Allders Award was inconsistent with the provisions of the NSW Anti-Discrimination Act 1977. It further found that the Award was silent on the subject of retirement age of employees.

In its 'decision' of 18 July 1985 the Tribunal, Ms K. Loder, Mr G. Suryn and Dr B. Thiering, found that Ms Anstee's employer did not dispute terminating her employment on her reaching 60. Nor did they dispute that, had she been a man, she would not have been terminated until age 65. The Tribunal concluded that Ms Anstee was discriminated against on the ground of her sex because she was treated less favourably than her employer would treat a man in the same circumstances. The Tribunal awarded damages of $31891.50, with $1000 for 'hurt, humiliation and injury to feelings' and the rest for loss of salary. The Tribunal rejected the view that Allders acted vindictively and concluded that it acted 'out of a misapprehension that the availability of a pension at age 60 for women justifies the existence of its discriminatory policy'.

The shock waves from this case led to substantial delays in the plans to include 'age' in the Act as grounds for discrimination. On the other hand there was little impact on the employment patterns of older women. It seemed they 'retired' at similar ages and similar rates before and after the case. This is not surprising since most people are either unaware of their rights under the law or are reluctant to exercise them.

A colleague reported the following case in a meeting discussing abuse of older people. He encountered a surprising 'blindness' to older people's needs in normal hospital routines. A sprightly 90-year-old woman had been living happily alone at home but arthritis had reduced her mobility. She was admitted to hospital for a difficult operation and while there the local Aged Care Assessment Team provided her with a list of nursing homes in the area. She had made no final plans about where she wanted to go. A day later, a Friday afternoon at 2.30 pm, her effects were packed by hospital staff, she was placed in an ambulance and despatched to a nursing home. However, she was not expected there and no bed was available. The woman had not been told where she was being sent in the ambulance, nor given any referral letter or discharge note. All she carried as evidence of hospital discharge was a paper bag containing seven days of medication. The possibility that she had been delivered to the wrong address was explored. It was 5 pm before the details of her hospital were discovered. By this time the woman was exhausted and distraught. The nursing home staff decided not to send her back to the hospital and found a temporary respite bed until a permanent one became available a week later. The geriatrician who observed this case feels that the hospital had regarded her more as an encumbrance, a package blocking a bed, than as a fully rational, decision-making person.

Structural blindness arises from unquestioned ageist assumptions about a person's ability or even right to make decisions. This neglect of evidence about a person's true mental capacity indicates bad practice and a failure to fulfil the 'duty of care'. Belated heartfelt apologies in such situations allow staff to excuse their behaviour as a one-off, correctable mistake, rather than a symptom of cultural blindness. The 'over-the-hill' assumptions seem to pervade Australian culture since so many individuals involved tend to be puzzled about how they make such mistakes. Simple adjustment of hospital procedures will not deal with the underlying problem here. More rigorous deconstruction of the events is needed if such mistakes are to be prevented in the future, since they emerge more often from structural blindness than from any intention to do harm. Regardless of how it is described, harm was done. In this case, for example, a competent woman was involuntarily incarcerated in an institution!

Structural blindness is the unwarranted neglect of the needs, beliefs and preferences of the elderly. It is not the product of demographic forces *per se*, but a result of inappropriate values and expectations and of the inability of bureaucratic systems to respond quickly enough to change. The system is blind when mismatches between needs and structures are made persistently yet identified only case by case, and ignored by those responsible.

Such cases are well known to various complaints bureaus. The Queensland Health Rights Commissioner has had to deal with cases like the neglect of the obvious needs of an older man both in hospital and in his neighbourhood. An elderly man fell in the alleyway outside his house and lay there for 20 hours before he was found. He was taken to hospital, x-rayed and told that nothing was wrong. The doctor and the nurses insisted that he walk on his injured leg. Later on when he continued to feel pain, his son took him back to hospital, where a new set of X-rays showed a fractured pelvis.[8] The issue here is not the error of assessment but the failure to listen to the older man's expressions of pain.

When the accumulating evidence shows consistent patterns but is repeatedly ignored or passed off as an 'isolated event', the system becomes brutal. Sometimes only a disastrous event attracting media attention will provoke a change. There may in some cases be a deliberate attempt to cover up individual problems, or a fear of losing face or power if mistakes are admitted. The situation is much worse if there is a long record of problems being brought to the attention of the relevant authorities but not resolved. Deliberate neglect of the need for change, in the face of mounting evidence, then amounts to structural brutality. A general lack of public accountability and access to information allows it to quietly reach crisis proportions. The mistreatment of vulnerable elderly people in nursing homes has received much public attention and has already been redressed by regulatory policies.

Commonwealth and State divisions constantly lead to complications and parallel systems that affect services. At another level people in positions of power, such as health professionals, can express their ageist attitudes in particularly brutal ways. The power of the professional, even when used abusively, is difficult to resist.

The Health Rights Commissioner hears many cases of professionals' abuse of older people. For example an older woman with severe arthritis, living on a pension, was advised by her orthopaedic surgeon to consider all options before proceeding with a hip replacement. The rheumatologist to whom she was referred told her that a rope around her neck would help her lose weight. During the consultation he constantly interrupted her, shouted at her to keep quiet and thumped his closed fist against the desk. His report to the referring GP described her presentation of symptoms as 'infantile, neurotic and intellectually immature'. He said that she would probably develop pelvic infection as a result of inability to maintain normal hygiene. While this is an extreme case it demonstrates how communication between powerful professionals and consumers can far exceed insensitivity and become brutally abusive.

Serious situations in specialist aged care facilities were also reported to the Health Rights Commissioner. An 85-year-old man who spoke no

English lived in a hostel owned by two doctors. As his dementia worsened, he sometimes wandered off for up to six hours at a time. His family believed that he needed specialised dementia care and arranged a place for him in a nursing home. The hostel owners who also provided his medical care would not sign the forms for nursing home admission, claiming that his condition did not warrant it. Shortly after this he wandered off again, fell and was not found for 20 hours. He was put in hospital but died a month later from pneumonia.

As well as neglect in health and aged care institutions, there is an ill-defined category of 'public neglect' where the consequences can also be brutal. Where resources are being wasted and services not provided to people at risk, some may legitimately claim to have been abused by the system. Consider an older person who falls, fractures a hip and dies lying on the floor at home because no emergency call service or home modification services were available in their area. Commonwealth/State divisions constantly lead to complications and parallel systems that have consequences for services.

Structural blindness or brutality, such as in the cases reviewed, is a consequence not just of individual failings but of social values misaligned with the aspirations of older people. Simplistic reactions to demographic changes do not even begin to approach these underlying problems. Vigorous deconstruction of existing practices and values is required by the groups of people involved in such cases. This becomes all the more important in an ageing society. The numbers of people distressed by such events does, however, increase with the growing numbers of older Australians.

Policy and structural blindness

Structural blindness has pervasive implications for policy. The most obvious response, and the one preferred by service provider groups, is 'more of the same' to meet expanded needs. More services are certainly required to meet greater needs. However, the strategy works only if services are doing the right things and if public money can be made available for expanding them. In any case, the expansion of services will not, in itself, solve the problems of structural blindness. As demand increases, so does the need for greater accountability to consumers.

Flexibility to expressed needs must also increase with demand. The attitude behind Henry Ford's now infamous phrase 'any colour, so long as it's black' is alive and well in the service industry. Older consumers in particular seldom have much say in processes that greatly affect their lives and well-being. This inflexibility of providers has been encouraged by a funding system that has always paid for new hospital admissions or new GP services but not homecare regardless of appropriateness or need. The absence of even the most basic management information—for example, on what outpatients receive—has also allowed bad practices to survive behind a veil of ignorance. Community services are not so liberally funded or hidden from public scrutiny as medical services are, but they can develop a similar capacity for inflexibility.

The marketing industry is starting to recognise the diversity and affluence of those over 50. In developing their approaches to this market, marketeers will use the latest and best technologies for measuring and evaluating demand patterns. They will reap the benefits of their commercial approach, or go under if it fails. They have already collected data on today's older consumers, and know that this group is better educated, better informed by media about various practices and consumer rights, more anxious about health risks, and more assertive in dealing with service providers.

When older people step outside the hospital or surgery, they find that they can order products to meet their needs. They can make detailed specifications for their new car that are sent to an overseas factory electronically, and the tailor-made product is delivered weeks later. This demand for individuality and manufacturers' recognition of the diversity of demand is characteristic of post-modern societies.

It is likely that greater numbers of older consumers, who are well aware that their tax dollars have already funded government programs, will demand a similar level of service from them. This will mean greater data collection and scrutiny of programs for efficiency. Structural inefficiency costs money and sometimes lives, and timescales for tolerance are shrinking in an on-line world.

These are some of the factors that will influence responses to the demand for more and better services. The days of paternalistic policy are numbered, and will give way to more consumer-focused systems in health and other areas. There has been a relatively recent emergence of new groupings of older people to address special interests in investment financial management, gender issues, education, housing and travel. Such groupings include Over Fifties Focus and Independent Retirees, Older Women's Network, U3A, Housing for the Age Action Group and Australian Seniors Network.

Older established national organisations like Council on the Ageing and Australian Pensioners and Superannuants Federation had long histories of significant advocacy and representation on a wide range of issues prior to the acknowledgment of ageing as a critical social issue. These organisations have evolved from a modernist welfare tradition to the active construction of a positive ageing movement.

The aims and vision statements of some of the newly emerging groups have a remarkable similarity to the older established groups, however their promotional material invites members to align with a particular sectional interest. Groups like Over Fifties Focus are emerging to give voice to their formerly unexpressed views and needs. These groups bring us back to the fact that not all ageing is 'bad news'.

Case 2: Over Fifties Focus—a group for Australians 50 years and over

Over Fifties Focus is a group open to people fifty years and over, living in Australia, who support the following aims:

- to enhance the quality of life of people 50-plus in Australia and to promote their dignity, rights and status as citizens;
- to encourage the representation of the views and needs of senior Australians;
- to provide and promote access to information, advisory and education services that enhance seniors' opportunities to exercise choice and further develop their potential;
- to promote opportunities whereby the skills and experience of people 50-plus are available to the community through volunteer and other services, particularly skills of an intergenerational nature; and
- to promote positive public attitudes to the ageing process and to senior Australians, and to remove barriers created by age discrimination, particularly in the area of employment.

The group, set up in March 1995, was sponsored by the Over 50s Investment Group in order to build on their financial foundations. The connection, however, does not mean that members also have to be members of the Investment Group. It attempts to give people over 50 a voice through an independent, non-profit organisation. Information can be obtained on Freecall 1800 555 150.

Other similar groups already exist or are being created all around Australia. For example, the Pensioners' and Superannuants' Associations are well known throughout Australia. Their national office phone number is (02) 9281 4566.

Funders, namely governments, are seeking means of dealing directly with consumers and their representatives and subsequently to contract providers to provide what people need. The funder-provider split is now the common parlance of service reforms. It reflects the power of the modern consumer as well as public sector interest in cost control. As both voters and service users, consumers can 'outflank' providers who don't respond to their needs and appeal directly to the government, who pays the bills. In a complex, diverse and information-rich post-modern society it is mandatory for policy reformers to consult directly with consumers about changes. This situation is a remarkable turn-around for consumers and a real challenge for both professionals and public officials.

Policy reviews have normally involved extensive consultation with consumer peak bodies as well as in more open groups, sometimes in remote areas as well as major cities. This process is laudable but even policy developed in consultation doesn't necessarily deal with structural blindness and brutality. These arise from ingrained assumptions about older people.[9] They require quite a different program of political action. Many of the groups who can deal with this have a more independent or antagonistic attitude to government and service providers. Policy-makers need to be closely connected to activist groups who exist to get under the skin of prejudicial cultures.

The origins of Australia's tendency to treat the aged with a 'benevolent paternalism' lie beneath the historical overlays of social welfare policies. The 19th century public and charitable support for the 'deserving' poor, excluding Aborigines and Asians, was replaced during the origins of nationhood by a universal rights movement. A wage earners' welfare state[10] for able-bodied non-Aborigines and non-Asians was developed on the premises of full employment with minimum income standards and basic welfare provisions. The preference was for immediate wages and high rates of home ownership versus enforced public saving and insurance for contingencies like dependency in old age. This produced a minimum set of provisions for the protection of older people against poverty and, more recently, lack of home and personal care. It was a system driven by the desire to provide the minimum material support for dependent elderly rather than to provide them with full access to citizenship. More recent developments in universal systems in Europe were blocked by the early arrival of pre-modern social welfare such as age pensions in Australia.

Re-routing older people from institutions to the community has not occurred on any significant scale until the last 10 years. Reforming nursing homes to make them more homelike environments (a reform sometimes called 'normalisation'), exclusively for people who could not be cared for at home, also began in stages through the 1980s. The expansion of community care began even more recently, in the late 1980s. The understanding of consumer services has only just begun with the introduction of Community Options and Community Aged Care packages into the aged care system (see Chapter 5). While these changes are in progress the next major battle is to accommodate older people's preferences in all areas of public policy.

But what has happened to the 'light on the hill'—the goal of social justice much vaunted by the Australian Labor Party and its supporters? While support for a 'safety net' remains strong, little effort has been made to address the underlying problems of the inequality of the distribution of health, wealth and employment.

Public provision for older people is wide-ranging, but economic rationalism now tends to dictate resistance to any proposals that involve greater costs. Given the tensions between consumers and bureaucrats it is perhaps ironic that only by forming active political associations with significant consumer groups can policy-makers struggle through intensely competitive political processes. Without this political support they will be knocked out by other powerful groups. Older consumers are not reaching out for the helping hand but are starting to storm the hill to demand their rights. Old inequalities remain but the social participation of the aged in decisions that affect their lives can be enhanced.

Every public conflict creates opportunities for resolution. Because Australia is a highly developed country with well established social programs and safety nets, we are better placed than most to respond to the challenges of an ageing society. Already some commercial interests are responding to the potential they see for attracting the retirement dollars of the rising tide of affluent old. Thirty years ago investment opportunities, over 50s housing and exercise classes were unheard of. We are exporting expertise to our Asian neighbours, and training is an expanding field. Medical technology and expertise in matters concerning aged care are well advanced, and in demand. One big 'sleeper' for consumer developments is the potential use of our growing superannuation funds for greater productivity and sustainability.

Another big potential gain would be to continue the development of more truly interactive policy-making and monitoring. Much progress has been made in developing consultation mechanisms, and in refining social research techniques that give policy-makers a more accurate outline of client needs. The push for greater participation in policies and programs is unlikely to fade. Combined with the development of multi-media technologies, which are already increasing demand for and potential access to government information, there is a good chance for more cost-effective and appropriate social services in the future.

The diversity and dynamism of post-modern societies demands new approaches to policy. Services have to be responsive to individuals and consequently must be more flexible and better coordinated. The all-knowing, all-powerful doctor, nurse or social worker is out of fashion. Professionals must cross disciplinary boundaries, respond to consumers and learn to act as entrepreneurs when seeking government contracts. With more education and access to information technologies, consumers have the potential to take control of services.

Conclusion

Demographic change is only one factor shaping the Australian reaction to population ageing. Social norms, institutional values and professional values are other key factors in the process. The clash between demographic movements and rigid social structures can lead to further conflict. The structures constraining older people and their aspirations are poorly fitting. They have to be remade to deal with the values of a post-modern culture and to make way for the new generations of older people.

We need to approach claims about ageing with a sceptical frame of mind. Like a lawyer defending the case for older people, we need to establish the accuracy of the facts and the credibility of witnesses. Many false claims are investigated in following chapters. These have been constructed carefully by particular interest groups and need to be vigorously deconstructed.

Once the facts are examined critically, it is clear that ageing presents challenges and opportunities for public policy. It will inevitably become part of a broader pattern of movement and development, some of whose elements are as yet unknown. It is encouraging to know that most of us now in the middle of our productive years will be neither destitute nor decrepit during our potentially long retirement years. It is, however, possible that our social structures will be too inflexible to meet our aspirations of citizenship. The remaining chapters examine the key issues for our ageing population and discuss where public policy is leading, and with what likely outcomes.

Notes

1 Fuchs, S. and Ward, S. 1994, 'What is deconstruction, and where and when does it take place? Making facts in science, building cases in law', *American Sociological Review*, 59: 481–500.
2 Turner, B.S. 1994, 'The postmodernisation of the life course: Towards a new social gerontology', *Australian Journal on Ageing*, 13, 109–11.
3 Laslett, P. 1977, *Family Life and Illicit Love in Earlier Generations. Essays in Historical Sociology*, Cambridge University Press, Cambridge.
4 Davison, G. 1993, *Old People in a Young Society: Towards a History of Ageing in Australia*, Lincoln Papers in Gerontology No. 22, November, Melbourne, pp. 2–3.
5 Ibid.
6 McCallum, J. 1982, 'Perspectives on the Transition from Work to Retirement'. *Australian Journal on Ageing*, 1(1): 27–35.
7 Riley, M.W. and Riley, J.W. Jr 1994, 'Structural lag: Past and future'. In M.W. Riley, R.L. Kahn and A. Foner (eds) *Age and structural lag: Society's failure to provide meaningful opportunities in work, family and leisure*, John Riley and Sons, New York, pp. 15–36.
8 Cases used in this study were provided by the Queensland Health Rights Commissioner and are used with permission.
9 McCallum, J. 1993a, '"De-Constructing" family care policy for the elderly', *Journal of Ageing and Social Policy*, 5: 1–6.
10 Castles, F.G. 1989, *Australian Public Policy and Economic Vulnerability: A Comparative and Historical Perspective*, Allen and Unwin, Sydney.

3

Safer than houses? A new age for retirement incomes

The idea of superannuation has been around for a long time, but with little relevance to most Australians. Until recently, home ownership and the Age Pension were all that most people expected for their later years, and these provided the minimum standard for their well-being. As an early provider of age pensions from 1909, the Australian pension system is a 'pre-modern' form lacking the universality of modern pension systems.[1,2]

> He was a happy and grateful man to receive 'a pension for life to the amount of two thirds of my accustomed salary' from his employer for 'retiring at a certain time of life'.
>
> > English writer Charles Lamb, in an essay titled 'The Superannuated Man' for the *London Magazine*, May 1825.

However, many assumptions about working life, and about the elderly, have changed profoundly since Charles Lamb wrote about 19th century retirement incomes. Aside from growing inequality in incomes and employment opportunities, probably the most dramatic change is that most women are now in the workforce, although with many lingering disadvantages compared with men. Equally important is the increase in standards of living and in life expectancy. As standards of living have gone up, years in the workforce have shrunk. A lengthy retirement is becoming more common, whether voluntary or not. These developments challenge the social entitlements of citizenship that have long characterised Australia as a 'wage earners' welfare state'.[3]

Changes to superannuation policy since the mid-1980s signal a shift towards an employment-related approach to retirement incomes. This is consistent with the policy shift outlined in Chapter 2, which gives individuals more responsibility for their welfare, and allows the publicly funded helping hand to pull back. Another important goal of superannuation policy is to increase national savings. Greater national savings, in the form of superannuation, will have a double impact on retirees: on their future personal income and on the national circumstances that will determine how far that money goes.

The new arrangements will affect each generation very differently. Since those already retired are generally unaffected, our attention in this chapter is on the baby boomers, born between the end of World War II and the 1960s, and the neXt generation, or Generation X, born from the 1970s onwards. The implications for both are profound. The recent expansion of superannuation to the masses certainly has the potential to become a great democratic achievement (Figure 3.1). In the longer term, many people should have a somewhat larger income than they would have received from the pension alone, and the burden on the public purse will diminish. However, there are concerns that

Figure 3.1 Percentage of employed people currently covered by superannuation

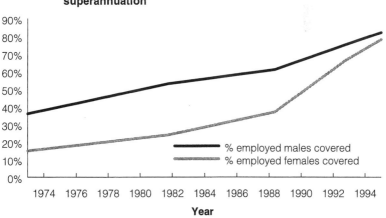

Source: Derived from ABS *Employment Benefits Australia* Cat. No. 6334.0 various years.

projected levels of replacement incomes will not be adequate to meet the rising expectations of many of the future elderly.

It is also widely recognised that these benefits will not be shared equally. Through the taxation system and the treatment of women, the new super system acts to entrench our present social divisions. As dependence on earnings-related superannuation increases, the gender gap in retirement incomes is likely to widen. Reforms were begun in 1995 to deal with these issues.

Another fundamental concern is the overall security of the funds, and the extent to which they are being used to create a strong and sustainable Australian economy. This also affects retirees unevenly, as low-income earners will depend more heavily on their super. The scandalous collapse in early 1995 of Barings, a major British merchant bank, took many British pensioners' savings with it. As the amount held in superfunds grows, so do demands for greater openness and accountability about the way the money is being managed. As with health care, this is part of the redefinition of responsible, participative citizenship which the new aged are bringing about. The context in which the current Australian retirement incomes system has evolved, and the likely impacts on our ageing society, are the subject of this chapter.

The way we were

A flat-rate means-tested Commonwealth age pension was introduced in 1909 to assist the poorest of the aged. This was a recognition that citizenship requires not only legal status, as a resident with rights to vote, but also adequate material well-being to exercise the benefits of this status. The Age Pension was available for men aged 65 and over, and for women aged over 60. At the time the average life expectancy for men was 59 (63 for women), so funding this pension out of general revenue was not likely to break the bank.

Australia and New Zealand were precocious welfare states. The early institution of flat-rate age pensions blocked options that appeared later in European countries—universal and earning-related retirement pensions. Our age pension has been cost-effective in providing a minimal level of well-being, appropriate to the prevailing sense of citizenship.

To appreciate the context at the time, it is worth noting that in 1906, over 80 per cent of men aged 65 and over (but almost no women) were still in paid employment.

Why were women given the pension at 60?

A quote from R. Teece, an actuary who testified before the 1906 Royal Commission on Old Age Pensions, captures the paternalistic flavour of the time:

Question: Is a woman, at the age of 60, as well able to earn her living in Australia as a man at the same age?

Teece: No.

Question: In that case, should a woman receive consideration that a man should not in granting the age pension?

Teece: Yes, I think she ought to get her pension at an earlier age. I would make it, say, five years earlier because I do not think a woman should be asked to earn her own livelihood at that age. I have a little chivalry.

An intrinsic caste system

Private companies began providing superannuation for a select group of employees from the 1840s, following the British model. Senior employees of banks and a few major insurance firms and utilities were given the opportunity to contribute and receive an annual pension upon their retirement. These were virtually all men. During and after World War II superannuation coverage grew to include more categories of workers in banks and major companies. This coincided with the mass entry of women into the long-term workforce.

Naturally the man who has nothing given him will receive a benevolence but a civil servant with a pension should never come to that—he would always have that income.

> Edgar Owen, a senior public official, speaking to the 1906 Royal Commission on Old Age Pensions.

Because women's incomes were still considered 'supplementary' rather than essential to household income, few women chose to participate in these superannuation schemes. Understandably, husbands' superannuation benefits became an area of dispute in divorce settlements. Current thinking recognises superannuation as a valuable joint matrimonial asset. Formal discrimination against women participating in super schemes took the form of lack of preservation, vesting and portability, and even compulsory sacking upon marriage (this applied in the Commonwealth public service until 1965). The modest security of our pension system acted as a buffer for women as the enormous structural shift involving them as wage earners, and led by the baby boomers, gained momentum.

Public sector employees were the Brahmin in this early caste system. They were much more likely to be covered by superannuation, and their schemes offered the most favourable conditions. They received relatively large payouts, often as lump sums, which were paid from unfunded schemes. Backed by the general revenue of a government, they could afford to be generous. The exclusion of married women from the Commonwealth public service, and the virtual absence of women in managerial positions, made women the 'untouchables' in this era of superannuation.

Some key terms:

vesting—retaining the employer's contribution and interest as part of your superannuation payout

portability—the ability to move your own and your employer's contributions when you change jobs

preservation—when your superannuation money remains 'locked up', or preserved until a minimum age, usually 55, even if the employee leaves and stops contributing

---

The Superannuation Guarantee Charge (SGC) sea change

By the late 1970s a dramatic growth in Australia's current account deficit had begun. Basically, this reflected how much more we were importing than exporting, and what sort of overseas debt bill we were running up as a consequence. The inescapable conclusion has been that we need to increase national savings, both individually and collectively. In addition, the government was concerned about the ageing population, in particular the large group of baby boomers, most of whom would depend on the Age Pension. Because the pension is funded from general revenue, the government feared that it would become an unacceptable burden by the turn of the next century. There were also doubts about the adequacy of the Age Pension as a 'replacement income'. The prospect of living on 25 per cent of average weekly earnings (the current level of the Age Pension), would seem like second-class citizenship for many baby boomers. Society has become both more complex and more affluent, with more items to replace and maintain, just to be part of the 'mainstream'.

Living at the fringe

Why isn't the Age Pension adequate any more? Although it is above the recognised poverty level, simple calculations reveal that it amounts to living on a pittance. We have made the following conservative estimates based on a single person who owns their home outright and relies completely on the Age Pension for income, along with various pensioner discounts. 'Extras' such as entertainment, owning a pet and operating a car are listed separately, to indicate how additional income from income-related superannuation or other sources might be allocated.

Table 3.1   Total income $8476 yearly

Basic living expenses (with generous estimate for pensioner discounts)		
electricity	$ 5 per week =	$ 250
gas	$ 5 per week =	$ 250
phone	$ 10 per week =	$ 500
food	$ 60 per week =	$ 3000
insurance on house and contents		$ 250
rates, water and general		$ 1200 (these vary by area)
clothes, personal hygiene,		
haircuts, shoes	$10 per week =	$ 500
	Minimum	$ 5950
Car		
registration	$ 450	
insurance	$ 350	
petrol, min $10 per week	$ 500	
		$ 1100
Pet min $5 per week		$ 250
Total with car plus pet	= $ 7300	
Remainder from $8476	= $ 1176	

Thus, a maximum of $22 per week is required to cover any repairs, maintenance or replacements for house, garden and car, all entertainment, holidays and hobbies, including dining out, magazines, newspapers, additional transport or phone calls, and all personal health needs, such as pharmaceuticals, physiotherapy, pathology or specialists' fees not covered by Medicare. With such a narrow margin, pensioners are forced to give up their cars and pets, progressively run down their assets and restrict their life-styles, possibly setting up a cycle of isolation, depression and costly ill health. It has been observed that pensioners will give up their Meals-on-Wheels service when the price increases by even $1. Would you want to live to this budget at any age?

The Australian Council of Trade Unions has been aware of these issues over the last two decades, and sought to avoid industrial strife yet win some gain for workers. One of the outcomes of the Accord between the ACTU and the Commonwealth Labor Party Government was a rapid increase in superannuation coverage in the late 1980s, while maintaining restraint on wage increases. This helped to keep inflation down while creating national savings to give workers a larger retirement income.

Part of the union agenda was to create industry funds that could be used productively to 'reconstruct' Australia and provide sustainable employment in the industries that had the highest union membership. Funds such as C+BUS, set up for the building industry, started to accumulate funds as a result of superannuation provisions written into awards.

But not all employers complied with award superannuation, and only 74 per cent of workers were covered by awards anyway. This was not enough to satisfy the need for greater national savings and higher replacement incomes. Thus, the Superannuation Guarantee Charge (SGC) was passed to bring all wage earners under the super umbrella as of July 1992. Universal provisions for super to cover low wage earners and those with broken work patterns were also considered necessary to provide for women.

The SGC brought in new standards to maximise employer compliance and provide for staged increases for employer contributions. The current target is an eventual 12 per cent of wages contributed annually to a superannuation fund, with 3 per cent from employees, and 9 per cent from the employer. This should be in place by the year 2000. Additional contributions from the federal government will supplement and provide incentives for lower-income super contributions.

Superannuation fits our pattern of a 'wage earners' welfare state', as defined by Frank Castles.[4] Australia has traditionally emphasised immediate wage gains and high home ownership over longer-term social insurance benefits. The new superannuation developments, achieved through arbitration, are largely employer-funded and offer workers a deferred benefit. This fits the pattern of central agreements between government and trade union peak bodies that has characterised Australian welfare.

As they fund the age pension through taxes, current workers are now also required to fund their own retirement by the system of forced savings in superannuation. Almost all Australians agree that older people deserve these payments, but historical changes mean that some are paying twice for retirement income—once for their parents and again for themselves.

Implications for the new aged

Although universal superannuation is meant to boost replacement incomes, it is likely to perpetuate, and even accentuate, persistent social divisions. It will link retirement incomes more closely to lifetime earnings, at a time when employment is less secure than ever for a growing number of workers. The irony is that the groups with the highest incomes and greatest earning capacity will benefit most from superannuation. The Age Pension will become a less than satisfactory safety net for those who have not provided for themselves through employment, and will create a pool of disgruntled elderly.

As Generation X matures and moves through life, they will find that their need to sustain hearty super contributions will influence life-style choices, such as taking time off for child rearing. Because their parents will mostly depend on the Age Pension, they will find themselves looking after them much as the middle-aged assist their elderly parents today. Both groups will have paid sizeable amounts into super funds.

Greater reliance on lifelong earning for retirement income places the onus on individuals to work hard and achieve their maximum income. However, the opportunity to earn has never been equal and, more important, the imbalance is growing. The substantial welfare reforms of successive Labor governments from the early 1980s have not impeded the increasing concentration of wealth, although they have softened the impact. Despite the cushioning effect of the welfare safety net, the gap between the highest and lowest income groups has widened dramatically.[5] Moreover, it is being perpetuated in neighbourhoods, with more and more jobs going to the richest groups. For every age group, the concentration of employed males in low socio-economic neighbourhoods is now lower than that of employed females in high socio-economic neighbourhoods. Education, long promoted as a great equaliser, is losing its ability to provide employment along with enlightenment.

As the following sections indicate, unwaged workers, most women and those on low incomes will continue to depend at least partly on the Age Pension well into the next century. The increased emphasis on earnings-related retirement income means that women will do well from super to the extent that they can approximate men's working lives and levels of income. This cuts out most of the baby boomers, and puts pressure on their daughters to lead busier and longer working lives.

Australia still has one of the most gender-segregated workforces in the developed world. Women's jobs cluster around the service industries and a few reasonably paid areas such as nursing and teaching. Women are also much more likely to work part-time, and to interrupt their working lives for parenting. These gender gaps are unlikely to close even during Generation X's working lives,[6] although a small but slowly expanding number of women on high incomes do very well from the new arrangements for superannuation.

To add insult to injury, the Commonwealth Government began a progressive policy of increasing women's eligibility for the Age Pension from 60 to 65 years. This further erodes women's retirement flexibility. Today's families have large numbers of single parents, and women paying off houses on one income. They will be under greater pressure to remain in full-time paid employment until the age of 65, assuming, of course, that they are not pushed out sooner. This trend, in turn, may have other spin-off effects, such as a greater demand for child care and aged care services, or even greater social problems if financial burdens prevent women (or men) from providing the parenting and supervision they would like to give.

Table 3.2 **Average weekly earnings of full-time adult non-managerial employees**

		1972	1978	1983	1987	1990	1991
Women	$	67.40	177.20	294.60	385.10	472.80	498.50
Men	$	97.80	216.70	358.00	465.00	574.80	595.60
Women's earnings as a % of men's	%	68.9	81.8	82.3	82.8	82.3	83.7

Source: ABS Average Weekly Earnings. Cat. No. 6202.0 plus historical data.

Women's total earnings, as a percentage of men's total earnings, are of course much lower because women are much more likely to work part-time. Many women looking forward to retirement after the turn of the century will find, perhaps to their surprise, that their super only 'tops up' the Age Pension, leaving them in fairly frugal circumstances. These women will wonder how, after running so hard and bearing for so long the dual banners of equal opportunity and family responsibilities, they remain at the bottom of the economic pecking order in old age. Those in good health and good spirits may well look for suitable means of exerting their rights of citizenship.

On the plus side for women, the new super funds are not discriminatory. The original Sex Discrimination Act allowed super schemes a blanket exemption from its operation, although it was intended that these exemptions would be removed. As of June 1993, changes to the discrimination provisions of the SDA mean that almost all discriminatory super provisions have been removed. These changes are intended to remove from super any remaining disadvantage or discrimination based on sex, marital status or pregnancy. In the past, areas of discrimination included access to superannuation, conditions and level of employer support and the resulting benefit. New funds or benefits set in place after 1 July 1994 must be non-discriminatory, although those who wish to maintain their present rights in a current discriminatory fund can do so.[7]

Not just some women, but all low wage earners will be disadvantaged by the tax structure of superannuation. Now that superannuation has been made compulsory for employers, and with the May 1995 budget for employees as well, the historic justification for tax concessions is weakened. Indirect pay through tax concessions on superannuation contributions has been called the most effective form of saving, especially for the highly paid, as they are in the best position to make the large tax-advantaged contributions. In terms of recurrent outlays, the additional budgetary cost of superannuation in tax cuts will not be matched by an equivalent fall in the cost of pensions until at least 2030.

For workers who earn less than a standard full-time wage, particularly if their working life is not continuous (i.e., most women), super becomes a series of small deposits to funds that charge a flat rate and are hard for individuals to track. A scheme introduced in July 1995 through the Australian Taxation Office will require the preservation of accounts so they can't be eaten away by administrative charges. There have also been many complaints about the fees charged to manage the funds. Some have suggested charging fees on a percentage rather than flat-rate basis, or on a performance basis.

It should also be emphasised that receiving the benefits from super-annuation depends on long-term employment. For most developed countries, it now seems unlikely that job growth will be able to keep up with the demand for employment, even though an increasing number of new jobs are part-time only, particularly those most commonly given to women. Restructuring for efficiency and competitiveness often means automation, and fewer workers. Steady immigration levels, mostly of young people, can make older workers less attractive to employers.

In this situation, many highly skilled, middle-aged workers can find themselves out of work, and many of them will have little or no accumulated superannuation to rely on. While the affluent old may well choose to retire early, many others will want or need to continue to earn a wage. As we will see in the final chapter, the diversity of the old will offer challenges and opportunities. Early retirement is increasing, but most of those who choose this option belong to a superannuation scheme.

Table 3.3 Age at retirement (percentages)

	1986			1992		
	Men	Women	Persons	Men	Women	Persons
Under 45	5.2	60.2	38.7	7.0	59.9	38.7
45–49	3.9	8.2	6.5	4.5	7.4	6.2
50–54	7.8	10.4	9.4	9.8	10.9	10.5
55–59	17.2	9.0	12.2	19.2	9.5	13.4
60–64	34.1	8.9	18.7	33.4	9.2	18.9
65–69	28.0	2.7	12.5	23.2	2.6	10.8
70 and over	3.8	0.7	1.9	2.9	0.5	1.4

Source: ABS *Retirement and Retirement Intentions* Labour Force Statistics. Cat. No. 6238.0.40.001.

Over this brief period, a slight convergence of men's and women's patterns can be seen, with an overall trend towards earlier retirement. Even so, since many males (but hardly any females) are still working after the age of 65, other aspects of security for their older years need to be firmly established in planning and policy. Encouraging and assisting middle-aged people to get into the housing market might be one way of preventing poverty among the aged. Fortunately, home ownership levels remain very high in Australia. The new aged will not be poverty-stricken, but they might not be as affluent as they would have hoped.

Table 3.4   1994 Housing Survey

All adults	
Home owners	42% of all households
Purchasers	28%
Renters	28%
Other	2%
65+	
Home owners	76%
Renters	16%
Other	8%

Source: ABS 1994 Housing Survey.

These developments may hasten the establishment of new structures and the revision of citizenship concepts along the lines of social participation rather than wealth and status. New views of citizenship emphasise social protection and interdependence with others. They expand 'work' to include any contribution to public or private welfare, whether or not it is paid. Although this concept was initially put forward by Bettina Cass in reference to increasing numbers of youthful unemployed, the argument carries over to an ageing society.[8] We are going to see a surge in the numbers of people middle-aged and older, healthy and willing, but not necessarily wealthy. If we can harness this abundant 'social capital' in ways that are both individually satisfying and constructive, we will be going a long way towards a graceful greying.

We will have to look at other ways of paying a 'social wage', ones that go beyond the extraction of labour for set tasks determined by economic principles. A quick look at any community gathering will reveal the substantial role played by mature people with a bit of time to spare. What a powerful engine for change and reform they could be if fully empowered to design cities, fix up policies and make improvements. Their potential contribution far exceeds conventional ideas of 'volunteer work'. This door of empowerment is already being pried open by many of today's busy older people, who are insisting on fuller disclosure on planning and policies. They are ready and able to act on the information they receive, and knowledgeable in many areas. Other pathways will evolve out of individual attempts to overcome the disadvantages of inadequate replacement incomes. We might see a 'Nimbinisation' of the elderly, bartering away and involved in creative cottage industries, unconcerned about the stock market or interest rates. Like their grandparents, they will learn to make do, but they will be better prepared.

Already, in the United States, an involvement in the 'informal' economy has become discernible among the elderly who are also poor or black.[9] Such inclinations towards the 'black' economy has already been mooted as a possible outcome of the growing inequalities in Australian society.[10] Hopefully, today's policy-makers, many of whom are now in the home stretch towards retirement, will actively encourage and pursue interpretations of social well-being and the 'common wealth' which protect individuals along with the tax base. The Community Information Project being tested by the Department of Social Security includes a project aimed at setting up bartering and LETS schemes, via the Internet.

The super industry—a monster in the making?

While some are busy feeding their muse or their chickens, others will be keeping an eye on the formal economy. It will certainly need watching, as most of us will have a lot at stake in the super funds. This is where the second great consequence of superannuation comes in: the overall security of the money and its use to sustain and develop our economy. A brief look at the overall structure of the super industry is appropriate here, to show how and why tomorrow's elderly will be taking a keen interest.

The government estimates that nearly 90 per cent of employees now have superannuation coverage. The amount of money invested in super-annuation funds has likewise grown exponentially, to over $200 billion as of mid 1995, growing by nearly $90 million per day. Such large quantities of money could greatly boost economic development. Clearly, the bet is on that most workers will see their super nest-egg grow. But unless concerns about the management and security of the funds are dealt with, and unless access to information about these matters is assured, the super industry may be somewhat of a gamble.

Such a huge pool of money is a magnet for the professional money managers. Several trade union officials have moved on to lucrative careers as fund managers, building on their experience with industry funds. Funds are generally used conservatively, for investment in a spread of stocks, bonds and property. A small but growing amount is being invested overseas where the growing economies of Asia, South America and Eastern Europe offer high returns.[11] Management of the funds is highly concentrated, with just five companies managing over 50 per cent of the money. The names are familiar, as they have long been important shapers of Australia's economy: AMP,

National Mutual, Banker's Trust, MLC, Westpac. In 1991, these companies were responsible for managing just over $100 billion of the total $190 billion invested in superannuation in Australia.[12]

One of the problems with such concentration of wealth is that, like the movements of sub-atomic particles, they are affected by being watched. The markets see the super fund investments and respond accordingly. This in turn, limits the flexibility and effectiveness of these funds. While the fund managers claim that they are protecting their contributors' money, in fact the returns on super funds are typically just equal to average mixed trust returns. Their dependence on movements of international currencies and the stock market means that they are vulnerable to unforeseen collapses or other such events.

Fund managers publish outlines of the sectors they have invested in and their returns as part of their annual information to contributors. However, details of transactions are not available, and huge losses can be concealed. A movement has started for contributors to have some say in the way their money is invested. For example, workers nearing retirement might choose more secure investments, with lower rates of return.

Table 3.5 Is our superannuation money being used to secure Australia's future?

	$ billion		
	Net debt	Current account deficit Proportion of GDP	Total superannuation assets
87–88	96	3.41%	95
88–89	117	5.06%	108
89–90	131	5.79%	124
90–91	142	4.05%	135
91–92	154	2.94%	154
92–93	167	3.63%	169
93–94	163	3.93%	182

Source: ABS *Public Sector Financial Assets and Liabilities.* Cat. No. 5513.0 plus Treasury data.

The accelerating accumulation of money in superannuation funds has not been adding to national savings, judging from the growth in our deficit or debt over this period. The current account deficit also responds more to the business cycle than to the growth in super-annuation assets. For the future, the Commonwealth Retirement Income Modelling Task Force estimated a net increase in national saving of one per cent of GDP by 2005. A 1995 Access Economics report estimated 8 per cent of GDP growth in savings by 2003–4. While this is a help, superannuation savings will not of themselves solve the current account deficit problems.

Your risk or theirs?

The money that both employer and employee contribute to a superannuation fund will grow or shrink in value, depending on the investments made. An important question for future beneficiaries is: How much can I count on receiving at retirement? This largely depends on what kind of fund you belong to:

- *Defined benefits funds* give a final payout which is a proportion of the employee's final average salary. In these schemes, the employer takes the risk. Not surprisingly, these schemes are mostly limited to government and major corporations, whose assets can always presumably cover payouts to beneficiaries.
- *Defined contributions* or *accumulation funds* specify how much both parties contribute, but final benefits depend on the returns to the investments. In this situation, the employee, or future retiree, takes the risk. These schemes are more common for smaller, less secure employers who cannot carry the risk of large future payouts.

Almost all the new schemes set up through the SGC are defined contributions, which avoid many of the tax complexities that defined benefit schemes are subject to.

The 1994 Report of the Review of Commonwealth Law Enforcement Arrangements,[13] in a section on the supervisors of Australia's Financial System that includes the Insurance and Superannuation Commission (ISC), notes that 'it does not appear that law enforcement interests generally are taken into consideration when these agencies perform their statutory duties'. Steps are now under way to improve information exchange between the Australian Federal Police and the ISC. The Report also notes that the ISC's importance to the law enforcement community is growing.

The new Superannuation Industry Supervision Act has strict auditing and reporting conditions. Trustees are also under greater legal obligations regarding the probity of their funds. Even so, it is practically a law of nature that crime follows money, and it seems inevitable that some unscrupulous person or organisation will find a way to take an illicit bite out of the luscious super cherry.

There are also concerns that even investment in blue-chip stocks may not be as productive as it could be. If a company with major super investments is operating destructively on the environment or building factories overseas, what true value does super money have there? The call has often been made for 'green' investments, or investments in a more sustainable set of sunrise industries that could free Australia from the shackles of the global economy.

Peter Drucker,[14] argues that the huge investment in superannuation means that the contributors have a substantial hold on the major companies and, through them, the economy. However, since workers do not even know what companies their money is invested in, or have any practical say in the decisions affecting them, this rings hollow. And since very few women are on trustee boards, they have little opportunity to voice any different perspective they might bring to the overall orientation of the funds.

Clearly, more responsibility for a secure retirement income is being placed on individuals, and the superannuation game is getting tougher and more complex. Decisions on whether to vest or roll-over become make or break chances for the future. In this situation, informed choice is vital. Yet finding out about super options and funds is frustratingly difficult. The Australian Consumer's Association says that access to accurate and complete information about superannuation is one of the concerns most often raised by older consumers.

The new SIS Act places much more emphasis on communication with fund members, and requirements for beneficiary representation on trustee boards should help open up the flow of information. Women are being encouraged to become fund trustees, although trustees generally tend to take a fairly passive approach. There is a trend to make these positions paid rather than honorary, which may focus more attention on the task. However, even when information about entitlements and options is available to members, details are usually scarce and members seldom have any say over how the money is invested. This situation may well become the next hot issue for consumer activism. It brings us back to the dual purpose of super: individual income support, and a stronger economy to ensure that quality of life is not compromised.

Conclusion

With so much at stake in super, it is certain that future retirees will be watching the super funds with some vigilance. As a fundamental issue for intergenerational equity, superannuation rivals population and the environment. As they 'storm the hill', the new aged will be insisting that systems be established for greater openness and participation in the only investment that may match the family home in importance to them.

Notes

1 Shaver, Sheila 1995, *Universality and Selectivity in Income Support: a Comparative Study in Social Citizenship*, Social Policy Research Centre Discussion Paper No. 58, May 1995, University of New South Wales, Sydney.
2 Shaver, Sheila, and Saunders, Peter 1995, *Two Papers on Citizenship and Basic Income*, Social Policy Research Centre Discussion Paper No. 55, April, University of New South Wales, Sydney.
3 Castles, F.G. 1989, *Australian Public Policy and Economic Vulnerability: A Comparative and Historical Perspective*, Allen and Unwin, Sydney.
4 Castles, *Australian Public Policy*.
5 Gregory, R. G and Hunter, B. 1995, 'The Macro Economy and the Growth of Ghettos and Urban Poverty in Australia', Discussion Paper No. 325, April. Centre for Economic Policy Research, Australian National University, Canberra.
6 EPAC 1994, *Women and Superannuation*, Background Paper No. 41.
7 Office of the Status of Women 1993, *Women-Shaping and Sharing the Future, The New National Agenda for Women 1993–2000*. Australian Government Publishing Service, Canberra.
8 Shaver and Saunders, *Two Papers on Citizenship*.
9 O'Reilly, Patrick and Caro, Francis 1994, 'Productive Ageing: An Overview of the Literature', *Journal of Ageing and Social Policy*, Vol. 6(3).
10 Gregory and Hunter, *The Macro Economy*.
11 Fletcher. Jennifer 1994, 'The Emerging Markets Gamble Pays Off'. *Superfunds*, Aug, p.41.
12 Shaw, Diana 1991, 'Ownership and Control in Industry-wide superannuation funds in Australia in the 1990s'. Paper at Evatt Foundation Conference on Superannuation, Sydney.
13 Australian Federal Police 1994, Report of the Review of Commonwealth Law Enforcement Arrangements.
14 Drucker, Peter 1976, *The Unseen Revolution*, William Heinemann, New York.

4

Ageing and health: The failures of success?

Not just the Australian population but all humanity is growing older. This is a great leap forward for health but is it also an impending financial crisis for the health system? As ever, the good news story is harder to sell to the media and the general public than the bad news about health and ageing. So we hear about older people dying before they progress through waiting lists for health services and about the severe rationing of health services threatened or already with us. Listening to the media alone is liable to create confusion about whether longer lives are a success or a failure of modern development!

In fact, both life span and health services for older people have improved remarkably. Our Medicare system provides extensive, low-cost and zero-cost health services and is widely accepted as an entitlement of Australian citizenship. Most countries in the world would 'give their back teeth' to have anywhere near the services older Australians have and at the same cost. Just as we managed without privatising education when the baby boomers were young, so the goal must now be to maintain good quality public health care throughout the period of population ageing. Thus we all need to take an interest to ensure that our health dollars are spent effectively and take into account changing needs as our society ages.

Younger people, the so-called Generation X, might not find much of relevance in this issue, just yet. However, the baby boomers, experiencing the first creaks of ageing and real or expected burdens from supporting their parents, are liable to focus much more on the social and economic aspects of health care. The ideal of a robust and active old age followed by sudden, painless death is, like winning Lotto, subject to chance events, to life-style choice as well as the game called genetics. Those for whom the dice have already been thrown, the current older population, have the first-hand experience of this issue and therefore the knowledge required for changing the system for oncoming generations. The baby boomers will be watching with intense interest as their parents move through the stages of disability and death, aware that acquiescing to cuts in services will rebound on them in the future.

The 'good news' of longer life is becoming tinged with fear for baby boomers and guilt for the elderly about the unintended consequences for health costs. Some interested parties predict that massive increases in funding will be necessary to satisfy the rapidly increasing demands from the aged in the near future. Some of these Cassandras in the private market have potential commercial interests in the so-called funding crisis. They argue for private sector investment to avoid the crisis but they shun regulation. We ask instead: are older people demanding all these services, or are providers imposing them on less powerful or ill-informed customers? We propose to critically examine the evidence for a crisis, and to 'deconstruct' some of the myths about old age and health.

The challenges of success

There can be no doubt that population ageing is one of the greatest achievements of the 20th century. Older people who remember some of the 'bad old days' are likely to be more appreciative of this than younger generations who have known nothing else but good health. In the last century rates of death in Australia were high—between 30 to 50 deaths per 1000 persons per year and much higher during periodic epidemics and disease outbreaks. The infectious and parasitic diseases were prevalent and childbirth was hazardous—all part of life not very long ago.

As the impact of these diseases causing death at young ages declined, degenerative diseases like heart disease, stroke and cancer became more prevalent.[1] Death rates stabilised to low rates of about 8 to 10 persons per 1000, about one-fifth of what they were last century and about where they are today. Prevalent diseases today tend to be chronic throughout extended life-spans rather than acute or fatal. In the most recent phase of the transition to longer lives, medical interventions and health promotion are lessening the impact of chronic diseases so that, somewhat paradoxically, people live longer periods of life with those diseases. New conditions can become substitutes for those we prevent. Avoiding a quick death from heart attack may leave the way open for the lingering 'living death' of dementia.

In an ageing society, death is no longer the major health adversary and the more significant threat is from chronic illness and disabling diseases that limit social participation and personal fulfilment. Some older people prefer to face death with appropriate support rather than to undergo 'heroic' and low-gain surgery. The high-tech virtuosity of the modern medical specialist may be considered by the older person as a degrading loss of control of their body and personal dignity. Older men may prefer to keep their prostates rather than go through surgery for a dubious gain and high risk of complications.

Health Rights Commission: Case 1

A 79-year-old man suffered surgical misadventure and his wife was told he was not expected to live. Nevertheless, she said, he was put on life support and had three strokes while he was on it. After that he was totally paralysed with a very poor quality of life. She and her children had opposed use of life support measures and had told the hospital that she was aware that her husband also would have refused had he been conscious.

The consequences of the transition in health cannot be dismissed as biological or demographic matters alone. They are historical and institutional and have to be worked through in the 'real politik' of the medical and health professions, in hospitals and health departments. The health implications of ageing are to do with inappropriate institutional structures and professional practices, not excessive use by older consumers.

Older people have been labelled as 'bed blockers', clogging up the system, but in fact there is evidence that older people's hospital stays have decreased faster than those of any other group. What is more, the provision of nursing homes and rehabilitation services offsets the typical mismatch of acute disease treatment for chronic disease in the elderly. Despite this all services are being asked to concentrate on treating faster those with highest need, and older people are most likely to find themselves still accused of bankrupting the health system.

Going for broke? The politics of aged health costs

It is obvious that population ageing has implications for health costs but are they of crisis proportions? Consultants writing for the private health industry, like Brent Walker of Tillinghast's (consultants specialising in advice to the private health industry), has written persuasively about a crisis in health care costs due to ageing. Walker's original paper appeared in 1991 at the same time as the New South Wales Government was replacing a public hospital with a private one in the town of Port Macquarie. The same issue made it onto the agenda of the Australian Health Ministers' Advisory Council (AHMAC) in that same year. The concerns about costs were genuine, but they were used with political purpose. The evidence produced in this debate was not complete: alternative readings of it, and contradictory evidence were not presented.

The evidence on older people's use of health services:

According to estimates made by the Australian Institute of Health and Welfare:[3]

- 8 out of 10 deaths now occur after age 60;
- half of all acute hospital beds in Australia are occupied by people over 60;
- people aged 65 years account for just over 10 per cent of the population but receive a third of the money spent on health care;
- the health expenditure per person is four times greater for those 65 and over than for those under 65;
- people aged 65+ consumed 34.7 per cent of hospital expenditure, 4.3 times the expenditures for those under 65;
- people aged 65+ consumed 35.3 per cent of pharmaceutical expenditures, 4.4 times the expenditure for those under 65.

The issue was again given prominence in the 1994 Economic Planning and Advisory Council analysis[2] of the cost implications of an ageing society. The projections were extravagantly taken forward 60 years, from 1991 to 2051, using demographic techniques. This assumes that the current average costs at any age will continue into the future. On this basis health care costs were projected to increase substantially, largely due to ageing. It was projected that people 65 and over would increase their share of the health budget from a third to half over the 60 years to 2051. The major concerns with the analysis are: the uncertainties of 60-year projections; the use of demographic methods for economic projections; and the contradictory evidence from historical studies.

The first critical question is whether cost increases due to ageing are more closely linked to the years of life remaining before death than to length of life from birth. Demographic projections assume that costs for different years from birth will continue into the future. The Australian Institute of Health and Welfare estimates show that about half the expenditure for people 75 years and over concerns the 1 in 10 who are within 2 years of death, so the other 9 out of 10 receive only half the health expenditures for this age group. The group within 2 years of death receive 16 times more than the average for the whole population whereas the rest of those 75 and over receive less than 3 times the average for the whole population.

In the longitudinal study of people in Dubbo born before 1930,[4] people who survived had eight times fewer hospital days than those who died over the first five years of the study. That is, the costs were mostly for those who died early in the study rather than for those who survived. For the youngest age group (60–69 years) the difference was a factor of 10 whereas for the oldest group (80+) the factor was 5 (Figure 4.1). This indicates the importance of preventing premature death in the younger elderly, as well as the fact that costs have more to do with time from death than with time from birth. Thus population ageing has minor cost implications because it shifts the high cost period to later ages without increasing the years over which high costs are incurred. This means that the projection methods used in the EPAC study made inappropriate assumptions.

Other historical evidence published by the Australian Institute of Health and Welfare[5] also appears to have been missed by authors of crisis scenarios. Between 1976 and 1986, from the Medibank to Medicare systems, the cost of services per person, adjusted for increases in Medical Benefits schedule fees, increased by 4 per cent per year. Despite these increases only a very small proportion, about 1 or 2 per cent of total cost increase, was attributable directly to ageing. Similar patterns in expenditures were observed for the more recent period for financial years 1984/85 to 1989/90 in Dr John Deeble's study for the National Health Strategy.[6]

Figure 4.1 Pattern of hospital use for dead vs survivors 60+ in Dubbo, Australia, 1988 to 1993

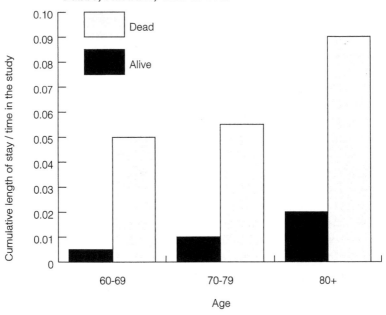

Source: Special calculations derived from McCallum et al 1994.

Looking to the future, evidence published by the National Health Strategy[7] in the early 1990s shows that total hospital admissions are expected to increase by a third, in the 15 years to 2001. Only 5 per cent of this increase is due to population ageing whereas 25 per cent is accounted for by population growth at all ages. The largest increase due to ageing is expected from 2011 with the ageing of the baby boomers. This is significant but it is still not the dominant factor in cost escalation. From the comprehensive evidence in a range of studies by different authors we must conclude that the numbers of older people are not a major factor in past increases nor in future projections of hospital costs. Of course the unexpected can happen but, at this stage, the evidence is strongly against a crisis in health costs due to ageing.

This result is consistent with Getzen's findings in an international study of health cost increases in 20 countries[8]. Cost increases in health were found to be attributable to rising per capita income, technological changes and other trend variables which affect people of all ages and so cannot be attributed to ageing. Getzen comments:

Extrapolation from higher health care costs per elderly person to higher national health care costs for a more elderly population suffers from a 'fallacy of composition' by assuming that what is true for the individual must also be true for the whole. The association between rapid population 'aging' 1960–1990 and rapid growth in health expenditures fails to control for other factors that were also increasing at the same time. (p. 98)

Since ageing is only a minor contributor to cost increases, the crisis claim is a distraction, sometimes deliberately made, from the more difficult task of realigning the health system with older people's needs. Blaming the aged for health costs puts them in double jeopardy: they are mistakenly accused of increasing costs, and their access to services is constrained because costs continue to rise.

Ageing addicts—polypharmacy in the elderly

Older peoples' use of medications provides a case in point for the cost problems of an ageing society and possible solutions. Balancing the negative story on costs is a positive story about saving public money by reducing the consumption of drugs as well as improving health outcomes.

National data[9] show that older people receiving the Age Pension receive 22 per cent of all prescribed drugs and 55 per cent of psychotropic drugs. The 10 per cent of the Australian population 65 years and over use 41 per cent of all sleeping pills and 26 per cent of all tranquillisers, sedatives and medicines for nervous conditions. The Pharmaceutical Benefits Scheme provides special access to people holding a pensioner's card if they are prescribed by a doctor.

A study of everyone aged 60+ in Dubbo[10] found that 18 per cent of men and 25 per cent of women were using three or more classes of prescription drugs. Self-prescribed (over the counter) medication rates involved 29 per cent of men and 44 per cent of women using two or more classes. Of those who were on multiple prescription drugs, 56 per cent of men and 76 per cent of women were also using multiple over the counter drugs. Some of these mixes were contra-indicated and should not have been used together. The word 'poly-pharmacy' has been coined to describe the concurrent use of multiple medications.

The tales of 'pharmaceutical restraint' of older people in nursing homes just don't go away despite new government standards of care in nursing homes and hostels. Eight out of ten nursing home residents receive at least one type of medication. It is calculated that in

1993 older patients in nursing homes in inner Sydney received double the medications received by similar patients in British nursing homes. Major tranquillisers were overused relative to the behavioural management of disruptive people who scream and wander. On the other hand, the doses of anti-depressants which could be justified on the evidence were typically low and ineffective and few residents with depression were given them. There are problems with both overuse and underuse of drugs in nursing homes and in the community.

Health Rights Commission: Case 2

A former nurse went into a nursing home as her dementia began to worsen but she insisted that she did not want to be sedated. Some of her demanding behaviour was labelled as troublesome and the nurses arranged for her GP to prescribe Serapax which was administered surreptitiously in her orange juice. She became suspicious and refused to drink it. Her family arranged a specialist assessment by a geriatrician who advised against using psychotropic drugs like Serapax and recommended behavioural therapies. Despite this the nursing home and the GP sought to defend their 'right' to sedate her against her will and specialist advice.

In a Melbourne teaching hospital over a 5-month period 28 per cent of admissions were drug-related and most of these were due to adverse drug reactions including the interaction of contraindicated drugs. But according to the national data, from another point of view, the older people admitted to hospital for drug-related reasons were taking nearly double the numbers of different medications compared to older people admitted for other reasons.

Estimates vary from a third to a half of people not correctly following their medication regimes, with even higher levels of non-compliance among the elderly. They take too many pills, as well as old drugs that they have stocked at home or obtained from friends. They tend to vary their prescriptions intentionally to minimise adverse effects and they follow friends' advice about what works, which indicates either lack of communication or lack of trust between patients and doctors.

There is also a hidden story about the efficacy of drugs for older people. Most drug trials have been conducted on younger, male populations to minimise risks of harm to participants and consequent litigation. However, most drugs are used by older people and women whose reactions have not been tested in trials. The trial results of older people differ from those of younger people due to physiological changes with age, greater numbers of interacting chronic conditions, and different social and economic circumstances. Hence better surveillance networks are needed to deal with the unpredicted consequences of this mismatch between trial evidence and actual use.

The priority is to get people off harmful or unnecessary drugs. A combination of pharmacist and physician teams in Australian nursing homes has been successful in identifying unnecessary drugs and discontinuing them without serious risk. As a result of consumer concerns about the abuse of medication by nursing home staff, the United States introduced legislation in 1990 prohibiting the use of antipsychotic drugs to manage screaming, anxiety, uncooperativeness and other conditions where these were the only symptoms. This reduced prescriptions by almost half. It is high time Australia took the same course of action.

Clearly the best option is not to have people on unnecessary medications in the first place and to take them off medications when they are no longer needed. There are other options, too. Aspirin has been proven at least as effective for arthritis and other conditions as the much more expensive NSAIDs and beta blockers which have more significant side effects. Why are older people coming out of hospitals and GPs' surgeries with prescriptions for NSAIDs and beta blockers instead of aspirin?

Perhaps the only effective way of introducing greater accountability would be to deduct from doctors' own salaries the extra cost of the more expensive and possibly less beneficial drugs and to deduct the costs of unnecessary prescriptions. The need for change is urgent because the uncontrolled growth in Pharmaceutical Benefit Scheme costs is crowding out other more urgent areas of health care for the aged.

Drug companies are major funders of all aspects of the medical industry—journals, conferences, travel research, and other less visible activities. Consumers need to become as sensitive to this as they are to tobacco advertising. The polypharmacy problem is a structural issue that can be addressed immediately by controlling pharmaceutical advertising and doctor training. Older people's behaviour is a secondary issue. The polypharmacy case shows that health costs are amenable to change and definitely manageable. Recommendations on how this might be achieved are set out in a policy document produced by the National Health and Medical Research Council.[11]

Health differentials—'his' or 'her' health?

Newly formed activist groups are beginning to focus attention on older women's health. Women's groups have worked hard for 20 years to convince women that their health needs are special and only poorly serviced by the health system. In a natural progression of interests, 1960s feminists are moving from women's health into discussions of old age. In France and in the USA Simone de Beauvoir and Betty Friedan have, respectively, written books on old age. Germaine Greer has written about menopause and the growing social 'invisibility' of women as they age. It is now hard to find a meeting on ageing without a special section on women. While this is a positive development, the absence of an equally powerful health lobby for men means that relatively much less attention is being given to older men's health needs. Is this justified, according to the evidence on health differentials? Indeed, is sex the major divide or is it ethnicity or race?

As already shown in Chapter 1, Aboriginal Australians are unlikely to survive to old age and this is a national scandal requiring a response in its own right. On the other hand ethnicity was generally an advantage for survival due to the 'healthy migrant' effect. Thus the issues for people of non-English-speaking background have more to do with service access and with the sensitivity demonstrated by the service system. But what of the gender differential: are women actually worse off than men in health at older ages?

Evidence on health differentials from the Australian Institute of Health and Welfare[12] shows that a boy born in 1992 expects to live 74.5 years whereas a girl expects to live 80.4. For the years 1985–7 men 65 and over had a death rate 61 per cent higher than that of older women and older men's death rates were higher than women's for all major causes:

- lung cancer—men 387 per cent higher;
- suicide—men 286 per cent higher;
- bronchitis/emphysema/asthma—men 196 per cent higher;
- motor vehicle accidents—men 92 per cent higher;
- ischaemic heart disease—men 69 per cent higher.

Although older men die sooner than older women do, the evidence is more complex for illnesses. Older men report fewer minor and recent illnesses, similar levels of chronic illness but more serious chronic illness than women. Older men report fewer days of reduced activity and fewer doctor visits than older women but more hospital episodes.

Prostate cancer

After rapid increases in recorded prevalence, prostate cancer has become the most common cancer in men in Australia but only the third most common as cause of death, after lung and colorectal cancer.

- The lifetime risk of developing prostate cancer is 1 in 23.
- The risk of dying of prostate cancer before age 75 years is 1 in 70.
- 85 per cent of prostate cancers occur in men 65+.

Prostate cancer is pre-eminently a disease of older men but it is not normally life-threatening. The causes of prostate cancer are not yet understood and age, race, country of residence and family history are so far the only accepted risk factors.

There is a growing perception that women's cancer screening is receiving priority over men's. However, 14 per cent of men without symptoms who are screened with the Prostate Specific Antigen (PSA) test will be positive but only 1 in 10 of these will have prostate cancer. There is considerable psychological distress associated with 'false' positive reports. There are also substantial adverse outcomes from the treatment of prostate cancer:

- after radical prostatectomy (surgical removal of the prostate) up to 40 per cent of patients have urinary incontinence, up to 70 per cent are impotent and 1 per cent die within 30 days;
- after radiation therapy up to 8 per cent have urinary incontinence and up to 40 per cent are impotent.

The Guidelines for Health Professionals from the Cancer Advisory Committee of the Australian Cancer Society and the Clinical Oncology Society of Australia state in *Cancer Forum* (vol 19, no 1, March 1995): 'There is insufficient evidence that men's health will be advanced through prostate cancer screening of asymptomatic men . . . The Society will maintain a watching brief and review its position annually.'

Evidence from *Cancer Forum*, Vol 19, No 1, March 1995.

In 1988 older men had a higher rate of disability than older women did.

For chronic illnesses, older men were significantly more likely to report cancers, diseases of the nervous system and sense organs, and diseases of the respiratory and digestive systems, for example:

- deafness—104 per cent more often;
- bronchitis/emphysema—73 per cent more often;
- back problems—55 per cent more often;
- hernia—45 per cent more often;
- heart disease—30 per cent more often.

Older women were more likely to report circulatory and genito-urinary system diseases, as well as:

- nerves/tension/emotional problems—50 per cent more often;
- headache—50 per cent more often;
- varicose veins—46 per cent more often;
  arthritis—26 per cent more often.

Not surprisingly, their poorer health outcomes make older men's risk factor status worse than that of women. Older men are 16 per cent more likely to be overweight or obese, 45 per cent more likely to be smokers and 46 per cent more likely to be risky drinkers. If these differentials in health and risk factors applied to Aboriginals or non-English-speaking migrants, they would attract far more attention than they do now.

Considering these statistics, it is difficult to support the claim of the women's health lobby that the health system has been designed by men, for men. Clearly, multiple factors are operating. At the heart of these differences in men's and women's health are complex interacting factors like genetics, physiological and hormonal differences, social roles and cultural behaviour patterns. The fact that females survive longer than males in developed human societies and in most animal species suggests that there is some biological basis to the difference. But biology has always been a convenient excuse for inaction on health matters that have been proven in the end to be modifiable and not merely biologically determined.

It's not hard to see how men's social and cultural roles have an adverse effect on their health. Typical male syndromes include avoidance of the feminine side of their nature, repressed emotional expression, pursuit of money and status, self-reliance, aggression and low investment in relationships. This male culture of hardiness, risk-taking and independence gives rise to quantifiable health risks, which are made worse by men's relative lack of social networks. The hard-line interpretation of the 'masculine' role seems maladaptive and anachronistic in our post-modern age, because it keeps men from observing and acknowledging their own illness and from seeking help and information. Attitudes may be changing slowly, as more men like Sir William Keys and Ronald Reagan go public about prostate cancer and Alzheimer's disease, respectively.

Of course, men don't just passively absorb these cultural messages. Traditional roles on many levels have been blurred, and many men pursue health as part of their other ambitions. On the other hand, many women are adopting male patterns and life-styles, putting them at risk from high stress, smoking and drinking. While health in old age is a men's issue it is also, through burdens of care, a women's issue. Just as men should take on responsibilities for housework so they should take on responsibility for their health. Thus, interest in older men's health should not be competitive since it concerns both men and women. Older women do not wish their spouses to die prematurely, leaving them widowed for long periods, nor see them lose their dignity through disabling illness requiring personal care.

The enterprise and efforts of women have done much to create an imbalance in health policies. There is a national women's health policy, a longitudinal study of women's health, ethnic and Aboriginal women's health policies, and a special research program for older women's health. There is a national focus on women's health, not just in the policies and research studies, but in special health centres, screening and other programs.

What is available for men? First steps are being taken in a men's health program in South Australia and a national men's health policy was announced by the Labor Party just before the 1996 Federal election, but there are few special programs for men's health despite overwhelming evidence of their gender-related health disadvantage. Separate and parallel health systems for men and women are economically unsustainable. Services need to adapt to be more gender-sensitive but not necessarily gender-specific. It is the health system in general that has to refocus and get back into harmony with our greying population.

Refocusing health services on older people's needs

Despite the increasing health costs the health system is not meeting the needs of older people. The extremes of the mismatch range from outright neglect to dangerous overservicing.

Health Rights Commission: Case 3

An 82-year-old man was admitted to hospital with a bladder infection. His family complained that as a result of low staffing levels he was not given proper nursing care and developed first a pressure sore and then gangrene. They also reported that he was not given adequate pain relief. Consequently he was transferred from the hospital to a hospice where he died infected with gangrene and septicaemia.

Health Rights Commission: Case 4

A depressed 70-year-old man had his shoulder fractured when the muscle relaxant administered for electro-convulsive therapy did not work. He then required a shoulder replacement operation. He was angry because he had consented to ECT only because he was threatened with regulation under the Mental Health Act if he didn't consent.

Ageing has been 'bio-medicalised', progressively defined as a medical 'problem' and treated with services funded from the public purse. This is evident from increasing rates of GP and specialist use and especially pathology, radiology and drug use. Ageing was once considered more as a life stage than an economic burden. Of course, in the past there was also no concept of retirement, either leisurely or otherwise. Dementia, probably restricted to the few who survived to experience it, was tolerated without special consideration. Although we may have made progress with medical treatments, we have taken only the first steps towards 'humanising' our treatment of the elderly.

We have consistent Australian and international evidence that what older people say about their health predicts their survival chances more accurately than complex and expensive bio-medical measures can. Older people who say their health is poor are about six times more likely to die than those who say their health is excellent.[13] These personal reports predict survival more accurately even after health and risk factors are integrated with sociodemographic factors in models. It should not be surprising that older people know their own condition! At the very least this should give us confidence in what older people say about their own health. It is desirable to create protocols for health professionals like GPs to deal with typical interactions with older people. Non-medical information, especially, is poorly dealt with in GP consultations.

The current service system is strongly biased towards the health provider, and obsessed with medical matters. The problem is that medical services are among the most expensive available and often inappropriate to older people's needs, as our example of polypharmacy showed. High-tech restorative care is designed mainly to prolong life and only secondarily to alleviate disability and suffering. A new 'geriatrically sensitive' medicine would first negotiate what services the older patient and their family need. This will take more account of patient goals and values, give more weight to palliative interventions than to life-maintaining ones, and do more to ameliorate the effects of chronic illness. At the very minimum, medical service should reduce the current rates of the iatrogenic consequences of health interventions for the elderly—that is, the incidence of falls taken by those on psychotropic medications and the adverse events experienced by those in hospital.

Not all the health concerns of older people need involve doctors. For example, emotional concerns are dealt with more appropriately by trained counsellors, feet problems by podiatrists, and musculoskeletal problems by physiotherapists. The problem is that most of the services are provided at full cost in the private market whereas medical services not requiring payment are available from bulk billing providers. Whoever treats older people needs a better understanding of older people's goals and values and should start with their expressed needs. Older people are discovering how they can control their medical treatment by writing advance directives expressing what they want and don't want done to them. This leads to potential gains for older people and in health costs.

Multiple chronic and acute disorders for older people, combined with complexity in diagnosis, places them at high risk in a poorly coordinated service system. Normally we think of the nursing home as the last stage of care coordination, one that provides all services in one place. However, it is not complete and older people can fall in the gaps. They may have difficulty finding what they should be getting or encounter service buck-passing. While not many older people fall into this situation, they are the high-cost service users. The prevailing rigid professional and program boundaries are, to say the least, not designed to benefit an older person. Services have to be made more flexible and specialist care coordinators may be needed for people with complex and intense needs. Our health system has become so rigid and complex for consumers that special assistance is needed to negotiate our way around it.

Health Rights Commission: Case 5

The pain suffered by a 99-year-old woman in a nursing home increased greatly during one weekend. Her daughter was told that the home had called her GP's number but his locum had refused to come because he did not know her. She was told that the home had called the GP again that night when the pain became unbearable but had still not managed to get a doctor. She died in the early hours of the morning after 18 hours of intense pain. Although the complaint was made against the GP for not attending, the nursing home file revealed that the first call had been for pain relief orders, not for a visit, and that they had not persisted when their later calls did not get through.

Options for reform

Many of today's elderly and more of tomorrow's will have experienced good health for most of their lives and will be used to having a wide choice and making informed decisions. They are unlikely to settle for finding themselves at the mercy of an insensitive, tightly controlled medical system when their health starts to fade. To keep costs down and to maintain a robust old age for as many and as long as possible, greater information and choice is essential.

Prevention and the encouragement of a 'use it or lose it' approach to old age are entitlements of as well as obligations on society and individuals. Thus, the rigorous evaluation of therapies and drugs must be publicly promoted. A shift away from high-cost, dignity-reducing medicine towards 'healthy ageing' policies will benefit all groups, except perhaps for those with a stake in increasing their market share of care. Better integration of medical, para-medical and social services will also achieve better outcomes and autonomy for older people. Two other avenues which will lead to better health outcomes and the cost containment of aged health services are: (1) funding for older people's health lobby groups; and (2) the wider distribution of information on clinical trials, patterns of use, home care options, medical insurance changes and much more. The older people's networks will pick up this information and run with it.

In summary the options for health service reform that have to be considered are:

- consumer-driven, not provider-driven services achieved by consumer and provider education;
- consultation protocols for service providers;
- critical guidelines for providers, emphasising best practice and reasonable limits—for example, for ordering diagnostic and invasive screening procedures and prescribing pharmaceuticals;
- evidence-based medicine relying on rigorous clinical trials and the economic assessment of all new and old procedures and drugs, with some of the costs borne by those who benefit;
- reductions in public support for the kind of health research and technology development that only marginally extends life without improving its quality, and a requirement that research proposals clearly demonstrate such benefits;
- a shift away from high-cost, dignity-reducing medicine towards 'healthy ageing' policies that emphasise prevention of disease and disability, and older people's self-help and autonomy; and
- increasing the efficiency and appropriateness of current care by providing more day surgery, more allied health services, better home support, and more community care.

Conclusions

We are only beginning to grasp the nettle of health policies for an ageing society. Population ageing has been promoted as a cost problem, and this trend has blocked the changes required for dealing with the real issues of reform of service structures. It is essential that older people are given voice in this process. This will allow the identification of 'win-win' options for policy reform, such as the reduction in the use of pharmaceuticals.

Evidence-based decisions are also critical. Current evidence does not support prostate cancer screening for men despite anxieties created by the media. Those who would gain from prostate cancer screening for older men, for example, are those who make test kits and provide procedures and treatments. The evidence indicates that older men would be worse off. Media pressure to create anxiety about this condition, or more generally about the health costs of ageing, has to be resisted.

We need to get the issue of the health costs of ageing into perspective. Health expenditures in Australia are 8 per cent of GDP compared to 9 per cent in Sweden and 12 per cent in the USA. Australia and the USA have about 11 per cent of the population aged 65 and over while Sweden has 18 per cent aged 65 and over. Clearly, population ageing has not had a disastrous impact on the total cost of health care in Sweden, and for the USA policy is more of an issue than demography.

Ageing does, however, present a problem: it concerns shaping a health policy that meets the needs of older people more closely and is within the means of individuals and the revenue base. There is, however, no crisis or imminent financial collapse that requires a rapid reaction. On the other hand longer lives are one of the great achievements of the 20th century and the Australian service system still rates, despite its deficiencies, as one of the best in the world.

Notes

Note: All cases used in this chapter are de-identified actual cases provided by the Qld Health Rights Commission and used with permission.

1 McCallum, J. 1990, 'Health: The Quality of Survival in Older Age', In Australian Institute of Health, *Australia's Health 1990*, Australian Government Publishing Service, Canberra.

2 Economic Planning and Advisory Council 1994, *Australia's Ageing Society*, EPAC, Canberra.

3 Goss, J. 1992, *An Economic Perspective on the Health Impact of the Ageing of the Australian Population in the 21st Century*, EPAC, Canberra.

4 McCallum, J., Simons, L., Simons, J. and Wilson, J. 1994, *Hospital and Home: A longitudinal study of hospital, residential and community service use by older people living in Dubbo, NSW*, NSW Office on Ageing Best Practice Paper No. 6, Sydney.

5 Barer, M., Nicoll, M., Diesendorf, M. and Harvey, R. 1990, 'From Medibank to Medicare. Trends in Australian medical care costs and use from 1976 to 1986', *Community Health Studies* 14: 8–18.

6 Deeble J. 1991, *Medical Services Through Medicare*, National Health Strategy Background Paper No. 2, Feb.

7 National Health Strategy 1991, *Hospital Services in Australia—Access and Financing*, Nat. Health Strategy, Issues Paper No. 2, Sep.

8 Getzen, T.E. 1991, 'Population Aging and the Growth of Health Expenditures', *Journal of Gerontology* 47(3): S98-S104.

9 National Health and Medical Research Council 1994, *Medication for the Older Person, Series of Clinical Management Problems for the Elderly No. 7*, AGPS, Canberra.

10 Simons, L.A., Tett, S., Simons, J., Lauchlan, R., McCallum, J., Friedlander, Y. and Powell, I. 1992, 'Multiple Medication Use in the Elderly: Use of prescription and non-prescription drugs in an Australian community setting', *Medical Journal of Australia*, 157: 242–6.

11 Nat. Health and Medical Research Council, *Medication for the Older Person.*

12 Mathers C. 1994, *Health Differentials among older Australians*, Australian Institute of Health and Welfare: Health Monitoring series No. 2, Canberra.

13 McCallum, J., Shadbolt, B., and Dong Wang 1994, 'Self-rated health and survival: A 7-year follow-up of Australian elderly', *American Journal of Public Health*, vol. 84, No. 7, pp. 1100–5.

5

Home versus homes: Aged care services for the new aged

Nothing conveys the negative image of dependent old age better than the old people's home. Images of the demented and disabled in wheelchairs living in decaying facilities flood the mind. Consequently, little causes older people more angst in discussions than nursing homes. Older people fear them because in the past, nursing homes meant poor quality care and abandonment by family and friends. It matters little that they have become high-quality care facilities and have been transformed from objects of ridicule to institutions with formal statements of residents' rights, heavily regulated by government. Memories carry the past into the present. This is particularly true for older migrants whose memories bear even more unsavoury pictures of the treatment of older people in other countries.

People who need institutional care because their behaviour is disturbed or because they are physically frail have little independence or self-determination. They cannot achieve their aspirations for citizenship without considerable support from others. This threat alone makes nursing home admission a negative expectation for many people. In the past it was the means of excluding inconvenient and embarrassing cases from normal social life. It is a challenge to Australian society to provide dignity and self-determination to the minority of dependent elderly among the aged. This is one extreme of the range of citizenship options for older Australians.

Aged care services have developed a broad range of options besides services provided in institutions such as hostels and nursing homes. They also involve a partnership with private households and informal social support, the dominant sources of community care. Formal aged care services normally refer to services delivered at home or in special long-stay institutions for the aged, rather than hospital services or primary medical care provided by GPs. Health services were discussed in the previous chapter but we shall consider them here in the context of community and residential services as part of the total aged care service package. While health and community services are separated in terms of program definition and funding, in practice they are closely connected. For example, home and community care services are provided to needy people after hospitalisation, and the responsibilities for care shift between programs. From the consumer point of view they are all servicing the one person regardless of who provides them.

Developments in aged care continually produce layers of new health and community systems one on top of another. This makes for an ever-increasing complexity of service systems and providers. In recent years, community health and domiciliary care centres were popular at least in some states, then the Home and Community Care program became the dominant system, and case management innovations such as Community Options were added to it. Rather than producing a new coordinated system, this has created a consumer nightmare of different services operating under different auspices with different organisational layers accumulated over time. Although the Home and Community Care system carried one title, it has always been a loose amalgam of former, separate service providers differing in tradition and cohesion from place to place. It is now opportune to loosen these historical but dysfunctional boundaries between service programs and deal with people's needs more holistically.

From the consumer point of view all these services require co-ordination in what some people call a 'seamless service system'. An authoritative assertion of this need was taken in the COAG *Communique*[1] signed by the Australian Heads of Government in April 1995. It proposed that the reform of the coordination of health and community services should become the highest priority for the near future. Health and community service costs have become so expensive that new regimes of control are continually created to deal with them. The proposals for aged care are not new. As far back as 1975 the Social Welfare Commission recommended reviewing coordination problems in aged care. Services to older people are, by nature, complex and geographically dispersed.

The final plank in the service system is the oldest and the most used: family and friends. It is a fact that informal support carries the dominant burden of care for the aged. As Chapter 6 demonstrates, the evidence is that care support is becoming increasingly difficult and costly for the carers. Even minor reductions in the willingness of that sector to contribute support could have major implications for the costs of care. It could come about through the pressures created by the numbers of dependent older people or through changes in carers' attitudes. Structural shifts occur either way but the consequences for policy would amount to the same. The oldest and most reliable form of support may turn out to be the most vulnerable.

A developmental perspective

We need a basic grasp of the history of aged care services to see what values they embody and what fears they hold for older people. Old Parliamentary Inquiry records are an accessible source showing how the long-term, chronic needs of the aged were handled in the early days of white settlement. The picture was grim. The destitute elderly were incarcerated in 'protective' asylums and offered only the most basic support. In NSW, inmates of government homes for the old grew from 2940 in 1890 to 5399 in 1900, almost doubling. The superintendent of the Liverpool Asylum reported numerous cases of relatives disowning their older family members and even changing their names to avoid filial responsibilities. The Melbourne Benevolent Asylum, which was largely dependent on charity for finances, grew from 1337 residents in 1891 to 3436 in 1897. The overspill population were incarcerated in Pentridge prison.[2] With this grim situation in the relatively recent past, is it any wonder that nursing homes still frighten many older people?

It is also interesting to note the deep historical roots of the image of the 'domestically useless older male'. In the early years of this century most of the inmates of old people's asylums in NSW were older men, many of them labourers without property or living relatives to care for them. In Australia and in Britain at this time, older women were more likely to be taken in by families as unpaid help, doing housework and childminding. Men were less sought after because they were regarded as domestically useless and were probably less willing to accept help because they assumed the male stereotype of hardiness and independence. The situation in contemporary nursing homes has the opposite sex bias: women now bear a higher risk of institutionalisation because of their longer life expectancy and capacity to outlive their spouses.

The old-style institutions which have now disappeared from Australia can still be seen in the residential and psycho-geriatric services currently available in Asian-Pacific developing countries such as

Manila, and even some in more affluent cities like Singapore and Kuala Lumpur. Poor-quality environments usually offer minimal custodial care, sometimes with militaristic regimens, in situations that are akin to imprisonment.

In the early stages of the development of aged care services, voluntary organisations with various religious and social philosophies took up the care of the dependent elderly. In Australia the Uniting Church has had a major role in caring for the aged, along with groups like the Red Cross and the Country Women's Associations. In Singapore where Buddhist groups run aged care facilities and in Indonesia where Moslem women's social organisations promote care, parallel developments occur.

At some point in the development of countries, modern, high-quality aged care services emerge from these sometimes depressing beginnings. The key factor distinguishing the new from the old is the emergence of public funding for and public regulation of the aged care industry. It is a fact of old age that most older people cannot afford the high costs of services, and the few who can afford them for a while may quickly find themselves impoverished by them. Regardless of whether or not they are economically well off, physical and mental vulnerability puts older people at risk of exploitation by rapacious providers. Thus the roles of public regulation and funding are both essential to aged care services.

On the other hand the weakness of a system totally run by government is that it risks inflexibility in service mix as well as high costs relative to private sector options. Some blending of public and private providers may therefore improve the system but the government appears to have remained dominant in most developed countries. In times of budgetary pressures and public 'compassion fatigue' it is important that the strong public commitment to providing high quality services to the very frail elderly is maintained. The interests of the current elderly are not in conflict with those of baby boomers or even 'Generation X' who may have to care for them and who have a significant interest in establishing satisfactory expressions of Australian citizenship before they reach their own old age.

The development of publicly supported aged care is by no means easy nor without resistance from established groups. The first impediment in developed societies is often a strong medical profession which seeks to control services to older people even though many of their needs do not require specialist medical intervention. The problem is that medical services are among the most expensive of all, and this naturally limits the amount that can be provided. This problem was carefully avoided in Australia. During the 1980s the medical profession was more concerned with the re-emergence of Medicare national health insurance than with aged care reforms. The proposals for reform were manoeuvred into the new system by progressive geriatricians and other sympathetic doctors who 'stacked' the key Australian Medical Association committees so that major reforms could pass with little resistance. The big change was to shift the responsibility for recommending people for admissions to nursing homes from GPs (with rubber-stamp approval by Commonwealth medical officers) to a system of comprehensive, multi-disciplinary assessment by Aged Care Assessment Teams. This improvement in the service but loss of power for GPs was achieved by adroit politics but without the explicit cooperation from most GPs. Consequently they were elbowed out of the new system and the price of this was that we are now struggling to re-incorporate GPs into the reformed aged care service system.

The medical profession has also shown that it has the power to obstruct the development of aged care in other countries of our region. In the 1990s in Japan the development of community aged care services is impeded by a powerful, wealthy medical profession with high social prestige and untrammelled autonomy in what they define as their work. They have fought against the development of community nursing, preferring to have all nursing under their control. Nursing stations run without doctors have begun to appear in the community and are a popular place of employment for nurses despite medical opposition. The international best practice response to needs of the aged appears to have prevailed, in the longer term, over narrow professional interests.

The Australian medical profession did not resist the development of institutional care because many doctors controlled or owned private facilities. The problem for government became one of cost escalation and regulation was the response. Since access to a totally private system is very limited and the maintenance of quality standards of care under conditions of profit-making is very difficult, the owners of nursing homes are now subjected to tight regulation as a condition of receiving government funds to operate. As we attempt to make health and aged care services more flexible and integrated, it may be time to relax some of the regulation confining the operations of institutions and to develop a focus on desired outcomes of care which can be achieved in different ways.

The second impediment to the development of aged care services is the lack of public support for the taxes required to fund welfare state services. Most developing societies have not reached social solidarity on these issues and tend to believe that private families can and should support their own members in old age. This thinking does allow a residual welfare system for childless and abandoned older people. With increasing proportions of dependent elderly and changes in women's availability for care, this system fails to meet the needs of the elderly and their carers. The cultural desirability of family support is not matched by the ability of families to provide it and public resources must be devoted to care of the aged. Japan has already reached such a state and the needs of families in other developed and ageing societies in Asia are converging with it.

The development of aged care services usually progresses from family support (or destitution), to institutions for the childless and destitute elderly. Shame usually accompanies the state of poverty or abandonment by family. These early-stage institutions do not cater for independence and offer only minimal care. Out of these unpromising beginnings grow the modern aged care services of a developed state with professionally trained workers and high-quality standards of service.

Once public resources are provided for aged care services, the 'caring' professions should be monitored to make sure the services don't serve them more than they serve consumers. Service providers and their organisations can maintain or create dependencies that reduce consumers' opportunities for full expression of citizenship. Services should be provided in ways that enhance the ability of older people to find their own resources and those of their families and friends. Even in the modern welfare state the elderly still tend to be defined in terms of what is done 'to' and 'for' them rather than by what they do for themselves and others. Concepts like 'care, kindness and dependency' prevail over more activist ideas such as partnership, equality and joint negotiation.

Institutional services

The official goal of the Commonwealth Aged Care Policy rejects ageist assumptions, namely: 'to enhance the independence and quality of life of the frail aged and their carers by providing a coherent framework of community and residential care, which makes available high quality and cost-effective services appropriate to assessed need'. The question is, to what extent is this vision achieved?

Chapter 1 noted that in 1971 there were about 1 million people aged 65 years and over, by 1991 it was about 2 million and by 2031 it will be about 5.2 million people. In 1995 only about 40 000 older Australians entered a nursing home and they stayed about two years on average. Not many people go into nursing homes but when they do, a high proportion of them have diagnosed dementia and most people die there. While nursing homes provide the full spectrum of care, hostels have been developed to provide the kind of services that do not involve intensive nursing care. There were only about 59 000 people living in hostels in 1995. Higher levels of assessed needs are required for nursing home admission, because the level of care provided there is greater than in hostels.

Whilst nursing homes are part of a system of 'long-term care' most people do not stay very long in care.[3] In a study of length of stay in Australian nursing homes conducted in 1995, it was found that around one in three stayed only one month and a quarter of these died. About half of people stayed 4 months or less. On the other hand about a half of total bed-days in nursing homes were accounted for by the 10 per cent of residents who stayed for 5 years or more. Thus despite most people having short stays, the average stay was 636 days, a bit less than 2 years. The careful use of assessment can delay admission for most people until they are very dependent and near death. However there remains a group of high-need people, such as those with dementia or difficult behaviours, who require long periods of expensive nursing home care.

Low admission rates and short stays for most residents are the consequence of the strict assessment and allocation of people to care options, according to their needs. This is carried out as at 1995 by 140 aged care assessment teams throughout all regions of Australia, forming a crucial pivot for coordination in the aged care system. If other types of care, for example pharmaceutical use or even general practice medicine, had the same thorough gatekeeping and advocacy roles there would be less over-servicing and more appropriate use of public resources.

The Australian aged care service system is highly regulated by Commonwealth Government planning ratios determining the level of provision of different types of services (see Table 5.1). Under this plan, tenders are sought for new beds in under-serviced areas, and other adequately serviced areas are held constant although some may have a growing population of elderly. There are concerns that these rules for the numbers of 70+ may be too rigid to take account of the further ageing of the elderly as discussed in Chapter 1. A shortage of residential care may occur at the turn of the century because of the rapidly increasing numbers of very old people. In particular policy-makers should take account of a potential shortage of nursing homes for high-dependency aged persons, most notably between 2006 to 2016.[4] The battles for more residential beds may have to be fought now by the baby boom generation to make adequate provision for their future.

Table 5.1   Ratios of beds provided per 1000 people 70 years and over

	1986	1994	Goal
Nursing home	67	52	40
Hostel	33	46	52.5
Total beds	100	98	92.5

Source: Stevenson, D. (1995)[5]

The other main area of government regulation is the requirement that minimum standards of care have to be met as a condition of Commonwealth Government funding.[5] There are 31 standards covering quality of care and quality of life outcomes for residents. The Australian approach to standards is to focus on outputs rather than on inputs or care service processes. This allows reasonable flexibility in responses to various needs, for example the needs of those with cognitive impairments or who are physically frail, or have different social and ethnic backgrounds. However, the extra step to assess the well-being or enhancement of quality of life of nursing home residents, which would be a true consumer outcome focus, has not yet been made.

The standards require, for example, that residents be encouraged to live their lives as they wish and to enjoy a range of social and recreational experiences. Amongst other things they require that: accommodation be home-like; that privacy and dignity be respected; that residents' health be maintained at the optimum level; and that the facilities and their practices be safe and free from risk or injury. The elderly in nursing homes and hostels are vulnerable. They may be unable to express themselves or too weak to resist unreasonable behaviour from staff. Hence government regulation is an essential requirement to protect their interests and to maintain their human dignity and quality of life.

The Outcomes Standards have a legislative basis for enforcement if that is necessary but persuasion is the first step in the process. Standards monitoring teams visit facilities regularly to assess their compliance with the 31 standards. If a nursing home does not meet standards, the first step is to encourage the home to comply. If the situation poses a serious risk or indicates persistently poor performance, the Commonwealth Department can give notice that it will impose financial sanctions unless standards improve. These range from withdrawing benefits for new residents or, at the other extreme, revoking the approval for funding. The proprietor may ask for a review of the decision through Standards Review Panels which have been set up in each state. In the 1993/94 financial year the panels disagreed with only one decision made by the Department. These changes represent remarkable improvements in maintaining the rights of the dependent aged compared to the incarceration practised at the turn of the century!

Evaluation studies indicate that the outcomes standards process achieves results comparable to those in the USA and UK systems but at a fraction of the cost.[6] There has also been an improvement in the standards of care for frail elderly nursing home and hostel residents. This has become most evident in the appearance of vacant beds in homes with poor performance standards. Before these standards were established, consumers and their families did not have the information they required to evaluate the quality of care available in different facilities.

Two forces of relatively equal value have limited the taste for institutional care for the aged in Australia. First, institutional facilities are costly, more costly than community care for those with less intense or complex needs. Second, most older people would rather live at home with family and friends than in institutions. These forces have created a policy change in aged care because less institutional care meets the interests of everyone involved—funders and consumers. The new technologies and methods of care that are challenging the old style of hospital care also have relevance to long-term care facilities. More can be done at home than ever before, provided the right services and technologies are available.

It is better to think of long-term care facilities in terms of the people who work in them than in the bricks and mortar they are made from. Aged care facilities are centres of expertise that can be provided in-house or delivered outside to intermediate care centres and homes. Institutional care has, in effect, exchanged bricks and mortar real estate for an aircraft carrier with flying squads delivering services to a range of other facilities and households out in the community. People with disturbed behaviour are still likely to need coordination of their care in one facility but, in the future, imaginative community options are possible for other users of nursing homes and hostels.

Shifting the balance to the community

The regulatory and planning controls on residential care emerged from problems that became evident in the system through the 1970s. Costs of care increased alarmingly due to uncapped government building subsidies and care reimbursements which provided incentives for costly service increases. Moreover the lack of community care support created perverse incentives for people to seek residential care when, with appropriate services, they could have been cared for adequately in the community.

The major initiative taken to redress this was the amalgamation and reorganisation of diverse community services into the Home and Community Care program, which aims to enhance people's independence in the community and avoid premature or inappropriate admission to long-term residential care. The Commonwealth provides 60 per cent of funds and each state or local government provides about 40 per cent (although this varies). Around 107 000 people received home and community care in 1994. Currently, consumers of HACC services receive about 2.65 services per person, but the number of services used is gradually increasing. The main services received are home help, home nursing, home meals and program information services.

Case management programs have been designed to shift the balance of care even further from institutions to the community. Community Options and Linkages programs cash out the costs of nursing home admissions and provide those funds to a case manager to do whatever that person needs to maintain them happily and safely in the community. This is an innovation designed to achieve citizenship for the new aged with care needs! Individual care providers realise that cleaning gutters or pruning roses may be as critical to maintaining an older person at home as providing them with a community nurse. No longer is it a case of 'any care so long as it's HACC'. A second range of cashing out options has been developed in the Community Aged Care Packages which are designed for people who are eligible for hostel care. About 7 of these were provided per 100 people aged 70+ in 1994. This means that planning ratios for nursing homes are now supplemented explicitly by packages of care available in the community. Community care has truly emerged from the 'poor law institutions' days to be more amenable to modern marketing systems that are appropriate for the new aged.

Donna McDowell, Director of the Bureau on Aging in Wisconsin, USA, has been associated with the Australian Community Options and case management developments over the last seven years. She reported a case that demonstrated clearly the new style of service delivery for older people. An older woman with dementia had been living in the community without apparent problems until she started defecating on her lawn and neighbours' gardens. This caused immediate community complaints to the aged care services who came to assess the woman.

Under the older style of services, she would have received medications, home services or, most likely, been placed in a nursing home. Instead of this, the Community Options case manager spent some time investigating her background and discovered that she had been raised in a rural area and was used to toileting outside the house. She decided to try an experiment. She surrounded the bathroom with raw timbers to make it look like an outhouse and built a timber box around the toilet to make it look like an old 'thunder box'. The older woman accepted the new toilet and stopped defecating outside. She was able to remain in the community until she died.

There are many issues of coordination and flexibility in the current mix of programs for older people. Different programs allow easier access than others—it costs nothing to see a bulk-billing GP whereas a copayment is required for community services, which can only be received after passing strict conditions. There is little established evidence on the outcome of either service by which the effectiveness of the intervention can be evaluated. The services of a specialist allied health professional are often more appropriate than those of a generalist GP. However, the older person normally has to pay for those in the private market instead of having them bulk-billed under Medicare or through hospitals. For example, an elderly diabetic should seek specialist footcare from a podiatrist to prevent limb amputation rather than visit a GP simply because the GP's service is covered by the medical benefits schedule. Similarly it may be much more appropriate to see a physiotherapist about arthritis than to go to a doctor.

On the other side of the service divide, people can learn to manage much more themselves instead of depending on health and community services. A local swimming pool opened at times exclusive to older people may provide, through hydrotherapy, a better health program than any current service. Rather than waiting for meals-on-wheels, groups of older people could share a taxi and go out to a reasonable restaurant for a meal. Consumer services can provide new and inexpensive options for the community care system.

The rationale for funding community care as an alternative to more expensive institutional care has natural limits. We are probably already at the point where the proportion of people in nursing home and hostels cannot be shifted further to the community. Those in institutional care are heavily dependent on it and about four out of five suffer from dementing illnesses and disturbed behaviour. Such people are best provided for in one facility where all their care can be coordinated for their intensive needs. Community care is no longer required to shift the balance away from nursing homes; it should be provided in its own right. This means a shift to funding for service interventions to benefit older people in terms of health or well-being. The diffuse nature of social needs will make this a difficult process but one that will parallel new developments in health services. Community care has established itself in a short period as a major plank in the service system providing social care to people assessed with social needs.

How aged care services work in Dubbo

Since 1987 a group of researchers have been studying everyone born before 1930 in Dubbo, NSW—that is, all those aged 60 and over. Dubbo is a large country town with a population of over 30 000 people and a proportion of elderly just slightly under the NSW average. Older people in Dubbo were similar in most ways to the rest of Australia's aged population. The same people were observed over a specified period to ascertain what factors affect various outcomes. Hospital, hostel, nursing home and Home and Community services appeared to be working as intended.[7, 8, 9]

Older people with the worst health had been directed to the most intensive service options. Older people admitted to hospital had a 7 times greater risk of dying and a 10 times greater risk of nursing home admission over 5 years compared to those not in hospital. Those who were discharged from hospital to a nursing home had 11 times greater risk of death compared to those who were sent home. About 80 per cent of nursing home residents had a diagnosis of dementia.

A series of analyses were conducted to see what factors predicted service use over a 5 year period. Hospitals were found to be responding to health needs, nursing homes to high levels of disability and HACC services to social needs and disability. The significant predictors of hospital use were ill-health, older age and being a male. By contrast, nursing home admission was predicted by older age and higher level of disability. Use of Home and Community Care services was predicted by living alone in one's home and higher levels of disability.

Access to services varied according to payment and gatekeeping systems. For example, GP services are bulk-billed under Medicare whereas HACC services are subject to assessment and copayments. In 12 weeks after hospital admission 78 per cent visited their GP, 24 per cent received some kind of HACC service and 8.4 per cent received two or more HACC service, 4 per cent received Occupational Therapy, 2 per cent received Physiotherapy and no-one received Podiatry services.

Hospital admission tended to interrupt continuous HACC service use rather than to initiate an older person's first contact with the HACC service system. All people who received Home Care when they came out of hospital had been clients of the service before they were admitted. It was a lower rate for Home Nursing because this is a service used to check on older people after hospital care. Most of these people did not continue to receive nursing care after one or two visits. This pattern of service use suggested a radical option for management. Home and Community Care service providers could be better placed to coordinate care for older people than hospitals or even doctors.

And now the problems

While the system generally manages to get appropriate services to the right people, it is a poorly coordinated mix of complex services.[10] It is organised around different providers and their organisational imperatives rather than around consumers or service users. Many services are unknown to consumers and information about services is generally about separate services, not about the whole service system. This becomes a problem not only for consumers but also for providers like GPs who are trying to make appropriate referrals. It is a system which seems to assume that consumers can work it all out for themselves. Sometimes this assumption and lack of information is mistaken for a way of allowing consumers independence of choice!

Although the system is generally successful, quite a few criticisms can be made about it. Because of constraints on costs, the poor coordination of services and inadequate information about them, consumers do not always get the services they need. The point at which people enter the service system (for example, on hospital discharge) can influence the types of services they receive more than their assessed needs.

Service boundaries are not only organisational but also derive from different funding sources and methods of funding. There is a bureaucratic interest in shifting costs for services between different departments and different levels of government, particularly the Commonwealth and the States. States have been cutting Accident, Emergency and Outpatient services and pushing them onto GPs who are Commonwealth-funded. This has little to do with fitting services to consumers' needs and everything to do with bureaucratic cost shifting.

The structural barriers to more effective consumer-oriented aged care services are byzantine in complexity. A modern industry is developing around coordination, with different government agencies and provider organisations intensely competing for 'a piece of the action'. It remains to be seen whether the flurry of activity in coordination does bring better and more fully integrated aged care.

A model for consumer-based services

The key challenge will be to coordinate primary health care in general practice and in aged care services. This will not be so difficult if the services can focus more on consumers. At this stage general practitioners prefer to act independently of the aged care service system. It will be difficult to break down the barriers dividing a disparate group of about 17 000 GPs with multiple organisations representing them, all with complex internal professional politics.

A suggested model of the complex relationships required for focusing services on consumers is shown in Figure 5.1. Consumers express needs to GPs or community aged care assessment teams and care plans responsive to the needs of the person and their family would be developed. Instead of the multiple points of entry and multiple assessments that operated in the mid-1990s, the community assessment teams will be holistic and multidisciplinary, providing information and care plans involving the whole health and aged care system. It is not so much a 'seamless' system as a system with well-sewn seams in the right places.

In this model regional community aged care boards take on the responsibility of purchasing services on behalf of government from service providers. Consumers need to be in positions of authority and supervision on the boards of purchasers of health and aged care services. The quality and responsiveness of services will be monitored through contracts and funding agreements specifying performance standards and service outcomes. Funders such as State and Commonwealth governments delegate responsibility to these boards. Through the system there may be sets of services for conditions like diabetes, and guidelines and service recommendations specified for particular categories of consumers.

Conclusion

The costs of complex, ill-coordinated systems of care are significant and becoming inappropriate for contemporary life-styles. Yet community services are still very important means of supplementing family support. For a family relying on two incomes to pay mortgages

Figure 5.1 A consumer-based aged care services model

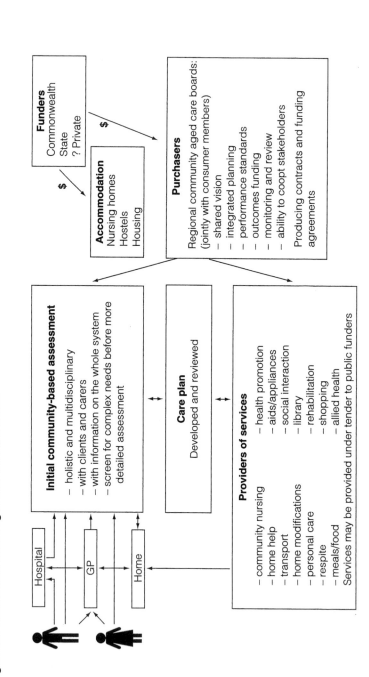

and school fees, it is a major sacrifice to stop work to care for a demented parent. Older spouses with more social life and leisure time may be unwilling to sacrifice their activities and health to care for a very dependent spouse. Collaborations between carers and public sector funders are required to keep carers adequately supported and rewarded. Australia is one of the few countries in the world to make carers a primary group for receiving Home and Community Care services.

To keep the service system alive for the new aged, the following changes are needed to accommodate structural shifts:

- aged care services must become consumer/carer driven rather than provider driven;
- greater flexibility between service types, including medical care, is required;
- since a 'seamless' service system is impossible, services should have 'well-sewn seams in the right places';
- services have to focus on consumer outcomes, not simply on administering services;
- carers have to be integrated carefully with the service system planning; and
- payments and services for carers must be improved.

New images of ageing require new service types. Social care provided by Home and Community Care services has now achieved a status in the community equal to that of primary medical care in its own area of influence. The role of the public sector is essential and must be maintained as the baby boom population reaches very old age. This will be best achieved by cementing the principle of access to community care as a right of Australian citizenship and by exploring innovative options for flexible and effective service.

Notes

1 Council of Australian Governments Meeting Communique, 11 April 1995, Canberra.
2 Davison, G. 1993, *Old People in a Young Society: Towards a History of Ageing in Australia*, Lincoln Papers in Gerontology No. 22, Melbourne.
3 Liu, Z. 1996, *Length of Stay in Australian Nursing Homes* Australian Institute of Health and Welfare, Canberra.
4 Gibson, D. and Liu, Z. 1995, 'Planning ratios and population growth: Will there be a shortfall in residential aged care by 2021?', *Australian Journal on Ageing* 14(2): 57–62.

5 Stevenson, D. 1995, 'Australia's Aged Care System'. In J. McCallum (ed.) *Export of Aged Care Services Training*, National Centre for Epidemiology and Population Health, Canberra, pp.49–60.

6 Braithwaite, J., Makkai, T., Braithwaite, V. and Gibson, D. 1993, *Raising the Standard Resident Centred Nursing Home Regulation in Australia*, AGPS, Canberra.

7 McCallum, J., Simons, L., Simons, J. and Wilson, J. 1994, *Hospital and Home: A Longitudinal Study of Hospital, Residential and Community Service Use by Older People Living in Dubbo, NSW*. Best Practice Paper No. 6, Office on Ageing, Social Policy Directorate, Sydney.

8 McCallum, J., Simons, L., Simons, J., Sadler, P. and Wilson, J. (1995) The continuum of care for older people, *Australian Health Review* 18(2): 40–55.

9 —— 'Patterns and costs of post-acute care: A longitudinal study of people 60+ in Dubbo NSW', *Australian Journal of Public Health*, Feb.

10 Dept Human Services and Health 1995, *The Efficiency and Effectiveness Review of the HACC Program*, AGPS, Canberra.

6

Carers come out! Family and community support of the aged

In 1993 Sydneysiders, and all Australians who heard the story, reacted with horror when a serviceman checking utilities stumbled onto the decomposed body of an elderly woman, Mavis Raines. Investigations revealed that she had died alone in her inner-Sydney 'semi' at least three years earlier, but no-one had noticed. The surviving family of Mavis Raines reported that she had asked them to keep away and that her solitary life was her choice. While we all appreciate the desire for privacy in our fast-paced, impersonal world, we worry about our society when the notion of a 'caring community' is so far from reality. Technology and media may allow us to be less dependent on face-to-face contact with other citizens for our social subsistence, but there is a lurking fear that total social isolation may not always be by choice.

Just when the memory of Mavis Raines was fading, the body of Clement Williams was discovered in south-west Sydney two years after he had died. Did he, too, just 'want to be alone?' We each have our own optimal mix of social support and solitude, and this may change as we age. But can we be sure that the types and levels of support and the interactions with others which could be so vital to sustaining us will be available in the future? Are we becoming too busy to recreate the caring society bequeathed to us by our parents?

The baby boomers are starting to face this dilemma with their parents, especially if they don't live nearby. Many elderly endure a quiet despair, in need of more help than is at hand. As the healthy early retirees of the future pass through the independence and stability of an active 'second adulthood', they will gradually become aware of how their greater frailty restricts their social and family networks. Yet it is

87

possible for public bodies and private families and groups, through foresight and good planning, to provide a seamless transition that will absorb the growing numbers of aged into communities without undue burdens. As we have seen with health care, there are already some cost-effective solutions, consistent with full citizenship concepts, which recognise individual needs yet encourage maximum participation and independence.

Many questions have to be considered when dealing with social isolation. Along with respect for individual rights, there is the question of who is responsible: the family, the local community or government services? A natural tension exists between the valuable role played by family, neighbours, churches and other agencies, and the right of older people to be 'free' from such 'do-gooders'. We also have to ask the fundamental question: Is contemporary society becoming less caring? How can we measure and analyse trends to get an 'objective' idea of how to proceed? From a more positive perspective, we have to acknowledge how much caring, mostly informal or unpaid, is done in the normal course of a working day in Australia. It is part of a normal life-cycle to go through times of caregiving and times of being cared for. This is true most obviously in families, but 'family' has become a nebulous term and caring extends beyond bloodlines. This chapter documents the extent and nature of caregiving in Australia and discusses how this vital activity fits into a framework for successful ageing.

Caregiving in historical perspective

The oldest form of insurance for old age is that of children and extended family relationships. In many developing countries, parents bear children because there are no alternative means of support in old age such as pensions and community support services. As these countries develop, they tend to supplement family care with public services and pensions. As a consequence, there is a decline in birth rates and, perhaps ironically, a shift to a more aged population.

Because it has been regarded as a private affair, family support has been relatively obscured from public scrutiny. It is managed within families and local communities—subject to the social norms of different cultures. In Japan, for example, it is typical for daughters-in-law to care for aged parents who live in the same house as themselves. This arrangement occurs rarely in Australia but is typical of north-east Asian societies. There it developed to allow viable portions of agricultural land to be retained in the family, rather than split up into small parcels. The land was inherited by the eldest son and it became his wife's responsibility to care for ageing parents. By contrast, in south-east Asian countries such as Thailand and Indonesia elderly parents are more likely to be cared for by their own daughters.

This is the normal expectation of Australian families, but our elderly tend not to live in the same house as their children and grandchildren. While about 7 out of 10 Japanese elderly (60 years and over) live in households consisting of grandparents, parents and children, fewer than 1 in 10 older Australians live in houses with their children and grand-children.[1] The Australian pattern has not changed much through this century because of the dislocation of families that is common in an immigrant society. Within specific migrant groups, however, the tradi-tional ethic of filial piety may be strongly supported despite the absence of extended family members due to migration. Thus daughters of first-generation Australian migrants may be reared without contact with grandparents and uncles, aunties and cousins, but later assume heavy burdens of care for ageing parents.

By contrast to these migrant families, 'mainstream' Australians are highly unlikely to live in the same house as their parents and prefer to arrange public support services for them rather than assume sole responsibility for care. Australians have held high expectations of public support through a benevolent welfare state, almost since Feder-ation when they retained much of the government involvement they had as a migrant colony of the British government.

Changing patterns

As in other aspects of Australian social life, everything is changing in family care. Women are staying on longer at school, more are seeking post-school qualifications and remaining in employment after they are married and have children. As discussed in Chapter 3, women are also remaining in the workforce longer, partly to supplement the Age Pen-sion, which is no longer considered adequate. The trend is particularly true for sole parents and divorced women. This diminishes the pool of people available to provide informal care and fundamentally alters the conditions under which people are prepared to take on care. It changes the nature of community life and reduces the numbers of people occupying a neighbourhood during a working week. On the other hand, governments everywhere are trying to constrain their welfare expendi-tures, and community services are low in the 'pecking order'.

Caregiving is caught in the pincers of a reduction of informal caregiving motivations and cuts to public supplementary support. For the baby boomers in particular, it is clear that the social largesse that provided them with schools in their youth and child care centres in their parenting years, will not be providing the same level of care for either their elderly parents, or later on, themselves. As an inevitable consequence of Australia's population ageing process, greater numbers of people living in the community will need care. At the same time, new policies are maintaining the nursing home type of patient longer in the community and older people are being discharged from hospital more quickly.

These forces raise serious concerns about how to maintain reliable informal care for the elderly. The major concern is that there could be a rapid growth in dependency on public services if ability and motivations to provide care in the community decline. Public sector cuts to community services could 'kill the goose that laid the golden egg'. What is needed is a fresh look at the role of carers and their relation to a much wider suite of services and policies. Changes in length of hospital stays or in stricter assessment for nursing home admissions all affect the informal support system. As with the related issue of health care, a more integrated approach has the best chance of solving several problems simultaneously.

The 'risk' of being a carer in Australia

The emergence of informal care as a policy issue has been driven largely by women's lobby groups and organised disability groups for whom family care was anything but 'invisible'. They pressured governments to make it an object of public scrutiny. In 1988 and again in 1993 a carer survey was added to the Australian Bureau of Statistics Disability Surveys. The 1993 survey[2] estimated that there were 2.2 million carers among 6.5 million Australian households. About 17.5 per cent of all Australian households included people involved in a caregiving relationship.

In 1993 there were 1 405 600 persons (51 per cent) 60 years and over with a disability and they accounted for 44 per cent of all disabled people. As age increased so did the need for help. Only 5.4 per cent of people aged 15 to 24 years with a disability needed help with at least one activity. For the 75+ group, 23.5 per cent of those with a disability needed help.

Definitions: Disability and handicap

Disability was defined by the 1993 ABS survey as the presence of one or more limitations, restrictions or impairments that lasted or were likely to last for six months or more, namely: loss of sight, loss of hearing, speech difficulties, blackouts, fits or loss of consciousness, slowness at learning or understanding, incomplete use of arms or fingers, difficulty gripping or holding small objects, incomplete use of feet or legs, nervous or emotional conditions, restriction in physical activities, work, disfigurement or deformity, long-term effects of head injury, stroke or any other brain damage, a mental illness requiring help or supervision, long-term conditions requiring treatment or medication, and any other restrictive condition.

A *handicap* was defined as a limitation on performing certain tasks associated with daily living. This limitation must involve disability and apply to one or more areas, such as self-care, mobility, verbal communication, schooling and employment. A profound handicap was defined as one for which personal help or supervision was always required. The total severity of the handicap was assessed according to the highest level of severity in any one of the areas of self-care, mobility or verbal communication.

> Australian Bureau of Statistics (1993) *Disability, Ageing and Carers Australia 1993*. Cat. No. 4430.0.

There were 577 500 principal carers aged 15 years and over who cared for a person with a handicap. Of these, 425 200 cared for a person in the same household and 152 300 cared for someone not living with them. Overall, 4.2 per cent of the Australian population 15 years and over were principal carers of a handicapped person, a rate higher than that of most diseases. The survey found that a total of 246 062 Australians with a profound handicap were living with other people, and 230 800 of these reported receiving informal help from a person in the household. These people were involved in constant, intense caregiving. An affluent society, which highly values personal independence, usually considers caring for a heavily dependent family member as a cost. While 'risk' is used in this section in the technical sense of 'probability', the term may also be appropriate in its common sense of suggesting a costly outcome! This will certainly not be true for all situations. Older spouses often find many rewards in the activities of giving care.

Carer profiles

According to the ABS survey, there are more women than men amongst the ranks of the carers and there are significant life-cycle patterns to caregiving demands, as follows:

- For those aged 15–24, the probability of caring was low but was mostly incurred by women. Most women were caring for a parent (5962) or a partner (3037).
- Of carers aged 25–44, most were women caring for children (53 625), parents (38 861) and partners (31 955). At these ages substantial numbers of men (19 583) begin to care for their partners.
- Most principal carers in the 45–59 age group are women caring for parents (54 538) or partners (33 170). Again, most male carers in this group are caring for partners (30 128).
- In the 60+ age group, caring for a partner becomes (for the first time) the main type of caregiving and men predominate in numbers of carers: 57 351 compared to 53 217 women.

Partners become less available for care as people age. Spouses accounted for about 90 per cent of carers of persons aged 60–69, and for 72 per cent of those aged 70+. Daughters account for less than a third of carers at the older ages, sons for about 5 per cent. This is markedly different from developing countries where adult children, not spouses, shoulder the main burdens of care.

Until the age of 60 women outnumber men as carers, and most of these are caring for children and parents. After age 60, caring for partners predominates, with slightly more men caring for women. The relative difference between men and women increases at older ages within the 60+ age group. Overall, women are more likely to be carers than men, but when partners need care in later life men become more fully represented among carers and in later life they are more likely to be carers than women.

Definition: Carer

Carers are defined by the 1993 ABS survey as people providing help (i.e. family, friends and neighbours) for categories of activities, namely: self-care (e.g. showering/bathing, dressing, eating/feeding, toileting, bladder/bowel control); mobility (e.g. getting out of the house, moving around in the house, moving from bed or chair); verbal communication (e.g. understanding someone who is known or unknown); health care (e.g. giving medication, dressing wounds, footcare); home help (e.g. washing, vacuuming, cleaning windows); home maintenance (e.g. changing light globes, doing the garden); meal preparation; financial management; writing letters; and transport (e.g. driving, shopping, public transport).

Principal carers are people aged 15 years or more providing the most informal care for self-care, mobility or verbal communication activities. The *main carer* is the person nominated by the recipient of care to provide the most informal care in all the above activities. Principal and main carers may or may not live with the person they care for.

Australian Bureau of Statistics (1993) *Disability, Ageing and Carers Australia 1993*. Cat. No. 4430.0.

There was a reaction to the 1988 ABS survey result when it was first reported, because it contradicted what some women's groups believed from their life experience: that there was a gender inequity in the burdens of caregiving. Understandably, the definition of a carer was criticised. For its 1988 Disability and Ageing survey, the first national carers survey, the ABS defined a caregiver as the sole or major caregiver who lived with a severely handicapped person and who was nominated by that person as the one who provided most of their care. By this definition, the care of older people is revealed as a matter of generational solidarity. It is provided mainly by spouses, and usually by female spouses, partly because older women are more likely than older men to be left without spouses. On the other hand, the 'domestically useless' male appeared well able to take on a caring role when required!

For the 1993 survey of Disability, Ageing and Carers[2], the Bureau broadened its much criticised 1988 definition of 'carer' (see box). It had been argued that the 1988 survey definition did not properly account for the women who provided intense care but were not necessarily co-resident with the handicapped older person. Two types of carers were now recognised, usually resident or not, and the main carer for each activity was distinguished from principal carer according to self-care, mobility, and verbal communication activities. The numbers of 'non-resident' principal carers identified by the broader definition were very low for the older age group. For 'principal carers of a usual resident' (the definition equivalent to that of the previous survey) the 1993 result indicated the same higher rate for male carers aged 65+, but not for those under 65.

It appears that stereotypes of men and women do not necessarily apply at older ages. After retirement men are not caught between family demands and work commitments. Anecdotal evidence also suggests that men have strong feelings of reciprocity when it comes to caring for wives. In later life they are happy to return the informal care their wives gave them during working life. For older people, caring may also provide a valued role at a time in life when entry into other socially valuable roles is highly restricted. In any case, rates of carers by gender tell only part of the story. Many older women do not have carers because their spouses have died. It is the greatest inequity to have spent most of one's life providing care to others and then to be denied it oneself later in life!

Having resolved the question of who provides care, with some surprising results, we need to ask what kind of support is provided. Carers assist with housework and home maintenance, transport, moving around, personal and health matters, meal preparation and verbal communication. In 1993 there were 1 106 900 people aged 60 and over living in households and needing help with at least one activity. The greatest need was for home maintenance (64.5 per cent) followed by transport (47.9 per cent) and home help (43.4 per cent). The group needing help was broader than the group who reported a disability.[3] About 7 out of 10 older persons needing help were identified as disabled. As well, older women who reported needing help outnumbered men. Women accounted for 72 per cent of all those needing help but for only 56 per cent of all persons 60 years or more living at home. Of people with no disability who reported a need for help, 85 per cent were females. These average patterns will be quite different for those caring for people with profound disabilities.

If we consider evidence from a more dependent older group, World War II veterans, an overall 7 per cent of Veterans Affairs clients had carers.[4] As for the older Australian population, 9 out of 10 carers of veterans were their spouses. The veterans serviced by the Department of Veterans Affairs had special areas of need typical of an older group. In the areas of personal care 13 per cent of all Veterans Affairs clients needed assistance with footcare while only 5 per cent of them needed help with any other matters such as bathing, medications and dressing. For more than 9 out of 10 clients with carers, their carer was their only source of help with foot care and most other kinds of personal needs. About 3 out of 4 of the carers who provided more than 4 hours of care per day had no-one to assist them. Around one-third of carers found that their service imposed many restrictions on their lives. Of those who were caring for someone who could not cope by themselves, just under half felt totally restricted and a further 10 per cent felt very restricted. While poor health was not necessarily due to coping alone, carers reported much worse health than would be expected for people of their same age and sex in Australia's general population, and 6 out of 10 carers reported being in poor or fair health compared to 4 out of 10 for people of similar characteristics in the general population.

Migrant carers

The population evidence on caring is only one part of the picture. In focus group studies of daughters caring for parents in first-generation Australian immigrant families,[5] it is possible to look in more detail at differences in values that affect caregiving. Generally speaking, migrant groups were much more willing to take on 'burdensome' care than were the Australian-born carers, who were much more likely to call on publicly supported services.

Family Group 1

A family with Italian origins was taking care of a severely demented mother who was capable only of taking a foetal position. This required 24-hour care by two daughters and a very aged father—the kind of care that would normally be provided, more or less free, in public nursing homes in Australia. One daughter, a mother of young children, gave care during the day. The other, a single working woman, did the weekends and evenings. They received some help from COASIT, the Italian welfare organisation, but these women felt severely burdened.

As the working daughter expressed it: 'I haven't got time to put my ear to a phone!' The daughters' care was provided with great love and some competence but it was not technically better than the high-quality care a specialist dementia facility could have given.

Family Group 2

In this case, a Greek extended family had sponsored the immigration of their mother after their father had died. They claimed that the dislocation of migration had caused severe dementia. It was almost certain that a previous, diagnosed condition had become prominent because of her move from a family situation, where it was accepted, to a new country. They moved their mother every fortnight to a different branch of the extended family, which greatly disoriented her but allowed them some respite from their duty of care. Women in this Greek–Australian community reported great cultural difficulty with coming to terms with nursing home admission. They reported leaving weeping husbands in the family vehicle outside nursing homes when they went to visit institutionalised parents. This lack of acceptance of modern aged care facilities among Greek Australians puts greater pressure on women carers than would have been the case if they had been able to use them without resistance from other family members.

Family Group 3

In a community of Vietnamese migrants, a question about whether the daughter carer had enough time to herself produced an entirely different response to that from other migrant groups. One carer said that she did have enough, but her description showed that the sense of personal space and time was quite different: 'Yes I can manage to have some time for myself. I can even manage to hop up and down at the same time as I keep an eye on mum. She cannot be by herself without me for an hour.' The Vietnamese daughter showed that she had almost no conception of personal space and time separate from family affairs. This attitude was the norm in the Vietnamese group.

Did this mean that Vietnamese–Australian women bore fewer psycho-logical costs from burdensome family care? The question about burdens of care may have to be asked in different ways for different cultures. Perhaps, in the absence of cultural modes of expression of personal burdens, the costs have been 'somatised' as physical complaints like headaches, pains and days off work. We cannot be sure whether responses from carers are stoic or honest. We can expect migrant groups to move more towards mainstream Australian values about institutional care since that happens in all other areas of migrant adjustment.

This erosion of migrants' traditional attitudes to care raises more general questions about whether men and women at the end of the 20th century are prepared to take on care burdens traditionally expected of them. In some groups this is clearly under challenge. As formal assistance moves further in the direction of cost-benefit trade-offs, so do individuals. However, the costs of a collapse of carer values and attitudes would be extreme, so policies are needed to maintain their participation in the care system. The overall picture of care for the aged, whether veterans or the general population, is more of an exchange between spouses than an intergenerational exchange between adult daughters or sons and parents.

On the issue of gender equity, men become more involved, as they age, with the care of disabled spouses, especially when they retire and are freed of the dilemmas of allocating time between home and work. Older women, however, are much more likely to be widowed and disabled without a co-resident caregiver than are older men. Over a lifetime women are much more likely to give care than to receive it. This unbalanced distribution of informal care arises from men marrying women younger than themselves and having lower survival rates than their wives. It leaves many older women dependent on the generosity of public service systems and family and community support. Women can be very resourceful in dealing with these situations.

At the lighter end of support there are adult children in full-time work who are now called on to deal more often with home maintenance and transport for their parents, and with unexpected emergencies. However, some ethnic Australian families and others are deeply involved in supporting very disabled parents. New surveys show that there are as many Australian workers with responsibilities for care of parents as there are with responsibility for care of young children.[6] The issue of 'family-friendly' workplaces concerns not only those with young children but also those with ageing parents. While child care has recognition in the workplace, the care of the aged has only recently been raised as an issue in workplace bargaining. This is a classic case of a mismatch between existing institutional structures and the expressed needs and aspirations of the population. We need to focus not only on the increasing numbers of older people but also on the values and practices that inhibit flows of care and support.

Older Women's Network (OWN)

The Older Women's Network is a community network run by and for older women. OWN organises workshops, information sessions, discussion groups and special events. It has developed a reputation as a consumer group. Its members are consulted on a wide range of issues. OWN has become well known as a theatre group performing political cabaret throughout NSW. Some exerpts from their cabaret songs follow:

On the Rocks
(Tune: In the Mood)
Cause we're older women

We're not over the hill
Being older women

Doesn't mean we're ill
Pills are not the 'cure-all'
There's much more to gain

Use it—don't lose it
Hang onto your brain

Mrs Everywoman
(Tune: Old MacDonald)
Mrs Everywoman was feeling low
EE I EE I OH
Life gets tough when you're short of dough
EE I EE I OH
So the doctor said
Take a Serepax here and a Valium there
You're ill—here's a pill

Australian Journal of Ageing, 1994, 13(1), p. 29.

OWN is committed to the belief that older women are the real experts in matters concerning their lives. It gives women the opportunity to get together and celebrate their lives in a caring environment. There are OWN groups in most Australian States and Territories and a rich variety of other groups for older people exist in the community, some with goals similar to those of OWN but few with the same radicalism.

Family and community caregiving at risk?

What do the numbers tell us about a potential crisis in caregiving? Don Rowland,[7] a demographer at the Australian National University, has pointed out that older people born before 1915 were much less likely to be married and, if married, more likely to be childless than older people born after 1915. This 'old' old age group of people are relatively deprived of children to care for them in old age. The 'younger' old, in contrast, are almost all married with two or more surviving children. These were the mothers and fathers of the baby boom children. They should reap the rewards of their investment if the baby boom becomes a 'carer boom'.

While numbers of caregivers do not indicate any impending crisis, there is still some cause for concern. The reliance of most dependent elderly on spouses for care means that population ageing is having a double impact. Both disabled older people and their carers are part of the rapidly ageing group who are at increasing risk of disability and handicap. The vulnerability of these carers implies that the next generation of carers, adult children, can become repsonsible for two older people rather than one. It will obviously be cost effective to support older carers so that their health does not decline as a consequence of burdens of care.

The dramatic changes in women's lives can affect their availability and inclination to care for their parents and, beyond spousal care, men have a poorer track record. Since most care of the aged is done by spouses, government polices for maintaining sick and disabled people at home longer may eventually jeopardise the older carer's health. In avoiding a single burden a double one may be created. This concern requires us to bring our ideas about and policies for caregiving into mainstream social and economic debate. There is also a vague but perhaps justified fear that contemporary Australian society is less caring or at least that it is harder to maintain supportive communities than ever before.

It is certainly a matter for concern when one in five Australian households are single-person units—an increase by 35 per cent over 10 years. The trend is largely due to ageing, with minor contributions from divorce, family breakdown and the diminished popularity of marriage. Who is home alone? In 1992 half of all people living alone were elderly and 7 out of 10 were women. Whereas over half of lone women tend to be widowed, half of lone men have never married at all, so more single men than women have no children at all.

While there may not be a crisis in aggregate caregiving, some groups may well be missing out. A recent ABS family survey found that men aged 70 years and over living alone spent an average 90 per cent of each week alone, not in contact with another person.[8] Their typical regular contacts were home and community care workers, for example on weekly visits, and neighbours (depending on their relationships with them). What is striking is that women in the same situation spent only about a third of their time alone. They are more likely to be in contact with family and friends, and more likely to initiate social contacts than men are. Even before widowhood, women have more intimate contacts with children and friends, than do married men. At least in this generation, married men largely depend on wives to make and maintain their social contacts. While partly self-inflicted, this tendency puts older single men at risk of social isolation. Despite the positive situation with caregiving in general, older people who do not have family or are isolated from them are a cause for concern. In developing countries, only the childless, single elderly are eligible for the full range of support services, where these are available. Australia has had no special category for such needs.

The risks of social isolation

Reviews of how survival is affected by social isolation (measured as a lack of social contacts) show that it is as great a health risk as smoking.[9] Despite this it is rare indeed to find social isolation as a target in national or state health policies. Investments in technologies, hospitals and medical salaries totally dominate other legitimate health interests. Social needs do not fit a medical model for services. There is no diseased or injured part of a body to be fixed. Nor is social isolation often a part of any health promotion campaign. Diet, exercise, smoking and even alcohol (which is often protective at older ages), are all frequently targeted but social isolation rarely gets into the picture. Lonely older people depend on home and community care providers like 'home help ladies' to provide social needs but this opportunity is gained only because they also have physical and mental health needs. Social need does rate as a factor in age care assessments but is not heavily weighted—people get HACC services because they are physically disabled or mentally ill. Thus despite the importance of older people's social needs, there is little avenue outside the family and the local community to satisfy those needs.

Government and community partnership in social support

The best publicised aspect of social support is caregiving but even carers have taken some time to establish a place in social policy. While caregiving was formerly regarded as entirely a private concern there was little chance of including it in policy thinking. The 1976 publication of the report *Dedication* by the NSW Council on the Ageing can be regarded as a landmark. The National Committee for International Women's Year sponsored the research. Its author, Clare Stephenson, later established the Carers Association of NSW. The Commonwealth Government commissioned further research in conjunction with the Poverty Inquiry which indirectly addressed these issues and kept them on the policy agenda.

As a diverse and over-burdened group, carers have neither the time nor even enough obvious common interests to present a united face to government. The women's movement did succeed in raising the profile of caregiving but policies tended to be handed down from 'on high' by a benevolent government. Carers Pensions and a benefit to compensate for caring for those who could be admitted to a nursing home (Domiciliary Nursing Care Benefit) were introduced in 1973. In 1993, outlays for Carers Pensions in 1993/94 were $121.3m and for DNCB they were $49.88m. The rates for these are derisory in comparison to wage rates but they do give some modest recognition to the costs of care. Many older carers, particularly those caring for spouses, are offended by or even resist the idea of being paid for fulfilling a moral duty.

Probably the natural extension of the idea of pensions and benefits is to pay wages to carers. Sweden pays carers at the rate of home helpers and allows for holidays and superannuation payments.[10] The Australian minimalist approach to pensions of all kinds is unlikely to allow a move to such generosity, at least in the short term. The experience in the mid-1990s with child care support may be instructive here. It was a relatively complicated process for families to apply for payments and many of the gains were clawed back in tax. Conservatives derided it as 'middle-class' welfare. The problems with a carer's wage in an Australian welfare culture raises similar issues, and the main problem is how to raise the revenue to pay for it. On the other hand, if economic pressures on carers lead to a widespread withdrawal of support, formal payment may become preferable to flow-on social costs. At present there are no satisfactory models that allow us to assess all factors and possible scenarios.

Choices for the future

The key issue is to understand what type of citizenship Australians are prepared to support, and what the minimum requirements are for social sustainability. It was previously argued that Australia developed a welfare state for workers, and based it on egalitarian principles. Some essential elements were basic family wages and minimum age pensions. This has been added to by universal schemes such as Medicare which allow nearly all older people to use medical services without restraint. It seems to matter little if people have these entitlements but are unable to enjoy them. For example, older people may become housebound and isolated, and may lose the social skills for participating actively in society. A full citizenship would allow people to exercise the choices that basic benefits are meant to secure. Programs for carers offering respite care, sitters and holidays, for example, provide such support.

While the home and community care program has the carer as a recipient of care, constraints on service costs mean that this is not always the most generous or available service. At present it is most responsive when an older person is seriously disabled and living at home, and when the carer's needs may take second place to those of the main recipient of care. This moves policy-makers into a more complex social model of care, one that does not seek as its primary goal a body to fix parts of or to rehabilitate to full function. The social model of care regards a person as a whole, connected to their community, and deals with that social group. This model is difficult to fit into simple assessment and cost control mechanisms.

Other options

A truly integrated approach to ageing would look at all the elements that contribute to well-being. It would recognise the continuum of life which, after the late blossom of 'second adulthood', inevitably leads to decline, whether rapid or gradual. A robust and resilient population depends on similarly robust systems, at all ages.

Consider this simple example. A stressed health care system that processes people at the most 'cost-effective' rate may not be able to resist new pressures. There is growing evidence that a rapid turnover of patients is linked to the spread of antibiotic-resistant bacteria such as MRSA which have become endemic in hospitals. In turn, elderly patients, whose immune systems are most susceptible, are most likely to fall prey to these bugs. This leads to extended stays in hospital, and much greater pressures on their carers during the rehabilitation stages. What would be the relative costs of less crowded hospitals, with more time for attention to infection prevention and early treatment?

Urban design offers many similar conundrums, where short-term savings create long-term expenses. A recent study in Canberra concluded that local shopping centres are no longer viable for the life-styles of the 90s. People, or rather those consumers who are most important to the market researchers, prefer the larger centres with wider choice and more facilities. However, older consumers may prefer smaller centres, with a less bewildering set of options. They may value ease of access more highly, and may be unable to travel to the big discount stores. Children or other carers may be called upon to assist, whereas in the past a gentle walk to the local chemist to get a script filled would meet some physical and social needs and help maintain independence. But younger shoppers, rushing about making consumer choices, hardly have time to think about the repercussions of their daily peregrinations. Nor should they be expected to, except as part of a thoughtful dialogue with city planners. Participation must mean more than merely acknowledging 'market forces.'

Transport is another major area of difficulty for the elderly and their carers. The younger group can still drive, but as they age, safety on the road becomes compromised by fading senses and reflexes. Urban densities, if allowed to increase without adequate public transport, also increase the dangers to young and old as traffic becomes busier. How comprehensively are such factors assessed when new housing is allowed in residential areas? Some of these issues are elaborated in Chapter 8, such as options for housing and the effect this could have on the carer's situation. Certainly, a great deal could be accomplished if we take a close look at how informal, de-medicalised mechanisms can be best supported and encouraged to thrive.

Conclusion

Our willingness to care for each other is probably one of our species' most enduring social characteristics. Only severe social and financial disincentives can erode this. However, pressures can lead traditional carers to withdraw their care if they are not relieved. Adjustments to support systems must be made to avoid this erosion.

Quite significant achievements for families have been achieved through policies directed at individuals, such as pensions and universal health insurance under Medicare. Carers' payments are a minor factor but alternative sources of help through formal services amount to a major initiative despite their limited rates of receipt. Linking informal carers into these formal systems is complex but necessary if we are to avoid eroding futher motivations for care.

Increasing numbers of Australians will be part of three-, four- or even five-generation families. They will, therefore, be involved with caring not just for older parents, aunts, uncles and disabled children but also for grandparents, great-grandparents, grandchildren and great-grandchildren. Social and demographic changes for families call for social policies promoting new roles, new relationships and new institutional arrangements for older Australians and their families, friends and neighbours. Policy-makers will have to become alert to the unintended consequences of outmoded policies and the costs of new public and private arrangements for care and support. The risks and potential costs of doing nothing about informal caregiving are too high to contemplate.

Notes

1 McCallum, J. 1995, 'Exporting aged care services to Asia: Regional trends and Australian responses', In J. McCallum (ed.) *Export of Aged Care Services Training*, National Centre for Epidemiology and Population Health, Canberra.

2 Australian Bureau of Statistics 1993, *Disability, Ageing and Carers*, ABS Cat. No. 4430.0, Canberra.

3 ABS 1990, *Carers of the Handicapped at Home*, ABS Cat. No. 4112.0, Canberra.

4 Federal Dept of Veterans' Affairs (undated), *Carers: Findings from the 1992 Health Survey of Clients and Carers*, Statistics section, Health Planning Branch, Canberra.

5 McCallum, J. and Gelfand, D. 1990, *Ethnic Women in the Middle. A Focus Group Study of Daughters Caring for Older Migrants in Australia*, National Centre for Epidemiology and Population Health, Canberra.

6 Russell, G. 1994, 'Workers with family responsibilities: adapting a wider family outlook', *Australian Journal on Ageing* 13(4): 161–3.

7 Rowland, D.T. 1991, *Ageing in Australia*, Longman Cheshire, Melbourne

8 ABS 1995, *Focus on Families. Family Life*, Cat. No. 44250, AGPS, Canberra.

9 House, J., S., Landis, K. R., Umberson, D. 1989, 'Social Relationships and Health'. *Science* 241: 540–4.

10 McCallum and Gelfand, *Ethnic Women in the Middle*.

7

Care for sale? Marketing services for the aged in Asia

Developing export markets for what we raise, manufacture or mine has long been seen as essential to a healthy Australian economy. Over the past decade education, and, to a lesser extent, medical technology, have also been export success stories. Australia occupies a special position as a highly developed country in a region where neighbouring Asian societies are ageing even more rapidly than ours. Now our history of developing expertise in aged care services is likely to become another important export earner. The government has already realised this. It sponsored a consultant's report in 1994[1] on opportunities and strategies for aged care exporting. The Australian Aged Care Export Network (AACE) was set up in 1995 after a series of developmental activities. This chapter outlines the opportunities and obstacles for Australian companies in the area of aged care services and infrastructure, drawing on examples of current activities in this exciting new field.

Cultural convergence

Global ads selling Coca-Cola are a prominent example of the trend towards a more homogenised, internationalised culture. The disappearance of whole language groups and traditional patterns of livelihood are sadder indicators. In Asia, rapid development and urbanisation are creating massive social change, similar to that experienced more gradually by Australia and other western countries after World War II. The wave of change that has accompanied the baby boomers throughout their lives has spread like a tsunami around the world. Asian women are entering the workforce in great numbers, many of them more career-conscious than their Australian sisters. Because the region is simultaneously experiencing rapid ageing, the social change this development brings is intensified, and is breaking down old family patterns of aged care and child care.

In some countries, for example China, vigorous birth control programs mean that ageing is actually preceding economic development. Regardless of the pace, improvements to standards of living and per capita incomes tend to increase the demands for services previously provided by individuals, mainly women. Governments in the region are acknowledging that they will need to support or supplement private enterprise efforts to meet growing social needs. Because Australia has had a long time to recognise and deal with these trends, we have solutions to offer which may need only some adjusting to suit Asian requirements. Even European countries are beginning to take notice of Australian aged care systems.

The spread of similar life-styles, eating, shopping and media habits means that the way our aged care services are structured (but not necessarily the way they are funded) will suit a wide range of situations overseas. One striking incidence of this came out during a focus group consisting of an Australian architect, an active service exporter, and elderly Japanese women.[2] When asked if they were happy to share toilets, they said that of course they would like private toilets, but they had never been offered the choice. It is very unlikely that any Japanese architect would have asked this question.

Of course, cultural convergence cuts both ways, and there is much that Australia can learn from its Asian neighbours. Our traditionally public services for the aged are shifting towards a more privatised approach, as with our retirement incomes policy. Asian entrepreneurial models and experience in providing these privatised services may well serve as models for organisations such as our superannuation funds in the future.

Some Australian aged care experts have already learned new ways of negotiating, having come up against firm bureaucratic and cultural obstacles more familiar to the hard-nosed financial sector. Overseas, some attitudes towards the aged, especially those of the staff who look after them, are initially shocking for consultants familiar with Australian standards. It is difficult for progressive gerontologists of the 1990s to recall a time when Australian attitudes to the aged were much harsher than we would like to admit. But we are getting in on ground level in Asia, and there will be a sharp learning curve for all parties.

Ageing trends in Asia

The ageing rate of the Asia Pacific region is unprecedented. The flagship economy, Japan, expects to move from 10 per cent aged 65+ in 1985 to 20 per cent in 2007, a span of just 22 years. Changes may be even faster in Hong Kong and Singapore. Economic development and ageing processes are being compacted into shorter time-frames than they are in other developed countries. In Australia the same change is expected to take 74 years and in France 115 years.[3]

In 1990 there were more than 84 million people 65 years and over in eastern Asian countries, including China and Japan, compared to 22 million aged 65+ in western Europe. There were even 49 million aged 65+ in Southern Asian countries including countries like India which we do not regard as aged. The numbers of Japanese 65 and over, about 17 million, already equals the entire population of Australia. The market for aged care expertise, from an Australian point of view, is unlimited.

Some grow older than others

A consistent by-product of economic development is an increase in life expectancy, with the advantage gradually going to women. Thus, we can predict a gradual feminisation of the aged. Perhaps this is because development brings improvements to basic health care and decreases in fertility, lowering women's childbearing risks. In underdeveloped countries like Bangladesh women still live 1.2 years less than men, whereas in developed economies like Japan they live 5.9 years longer.[4,5] A rapid increase in the numbers of very old is also expected. In Japan in 1990, 20 per cent of those aged 65+ were aged 80 years and over. This is expected to increase to 35 per cent in 2025.[6]

Another consequence of rapid change is that life expectancy in any current year becomes a poor guide to the real life expectancy of any birth cohort. Each cohort will live longer than the current death rates predict, as factors determining life expectancy are changing more quickly than the demographers can take into account.

Ageing at the oldest ages is more acute in the East Asian countries than in developed countries and it favours women more than men. This points to a convergence of demographics, with developed countries leading the way. In Australia the feminisation of the aged is well under way, and our experience in dealing with this gives us a relative advantage over many Asian societies, who are ill-equipped to deal with it. However, over-extrapolation may be unwise. In Australia, men's

Figure 7.1 Percentage increase in elderly population: 1990–2025

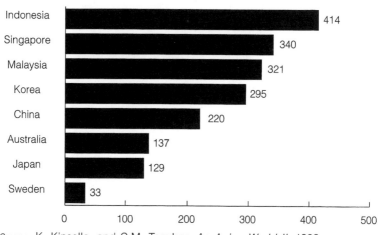

Source: K. Kinsella, and C.M. Taeuber, *An Aging World II*, 1993.

death rates are now improving more than women's. Is this the long-term cost of women's economic equality?

The golden period

Dependency ratios are useful but crude demographic indicators of how ageing affects family and social support systems. As the proportion of those aged 65+ to those of working age (15–64) increases, so does the pressure on the productive workforce to provide the resources to maintain the elderly. In an ageing society, the proportion of dependent young is dropping at the same time, softening the impact on social infrastructure. At different points in time for different countries, pro-portions of young and old dependent cross over. In China, with slow ageing, this won't happen until 2045. This crossover point is sometimes called the 'golden period', when it is prudent to invest in systems for aged care like pensions, health insurance and facilities before acute ageing puts extreme pressures on budgets.

Social support implications

The concept of cultural and demographic convergence can give us some idea of where Asia may be heading in the longer term. However, we need a much deeper understanding of the substantial cultural and

Figure 7.2: Percentage change in death rates by age and sex: 1977–87

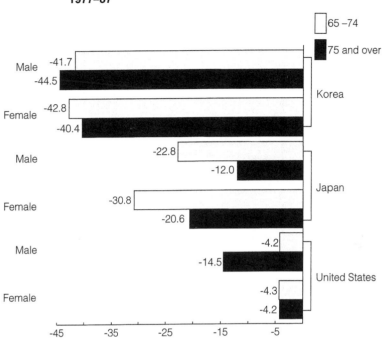

Source: K. Kinsella and C.M. Taeuber *An Aging World II,* 1993

political differences between Australia and Asia, within the region itself. Then we can see how Australia can capitalise on its 'head start' in dealing with ageing issues.

Living arrangements

In developing countries families are more likely to live in multiple-generation households, and to provide various forms of help, than developed countries are. Generally, family support is necessary, expected and available, for the care of young children and the elderly. Living alone is less socially acceptable and less possible. In many cultures it is considered a happy solution when the elderly are able to look after the young including their adult children and grandchildren.

As countries develop, young parents and the elderly tend to live separately. Women adopt Western working patterns, and fertility rates

Figure 7.3 Female labour force participation rates—Singapore

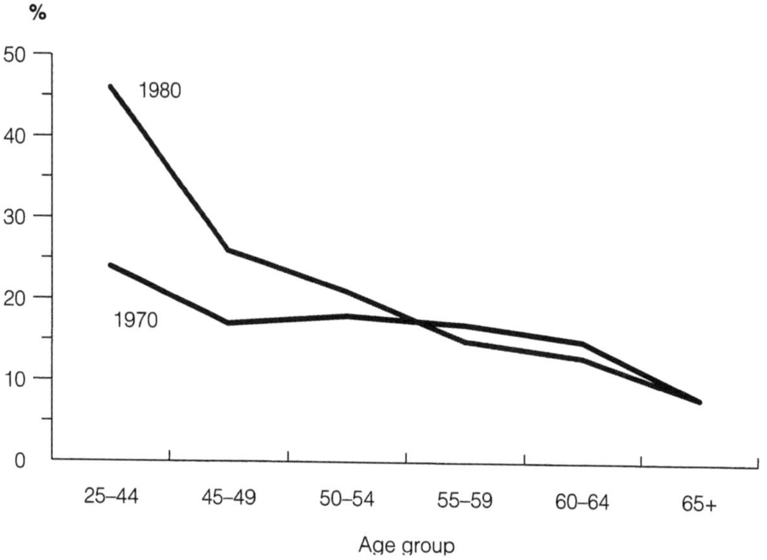

Age group

Source: K. Kinsella and C.M. Taeuber, *An Aging World II*, 1993

drop, so that fewer families need to live together. Women also become less available for the long-term care of the aged.

This developed country pattern is often interpreted by Asian observers as an abandonment of the elderly. There is a genuine concern that Western influences are eroding traditional filial piety. Most Asian countries have enacted legislation enforcing family support of the aged—Taiwan, Thailand, China and Singapore have, for example. In countries like Thailand elderly widows have the right to sue for return of property if they are not cared for by their families.

Living alone in a society where public support is unavailable can mean vulnerability for the aged. The numbers living alone in different countries reveal the following:[7]

- the proportions of older people living alone is considerably higher in more developed countries than in those less developed;
- the levels of people living alone rise with age to 85 years then decline;
- the percentage of women living alone is considerably higher than it is for men;
- over time the proportions of both men and women living alone increases.

There is a positive side to living alone, even for the most elderly. When development is accompanied by a rise in living standards, more people choose independent living. For the elderly, it may pose a risk if social and physical needs are not met. In some places, such as rural Thailand, one compromise is for the elderly to live in separate dwellings, but as part of the same compound. The introduction of the concept of 'nursing' homes or hostels in such a culture represents a significant break with traditional patterns of aged care. However, consultants working in Asian countries with a significant middle-class population report that there is a growing demand from these groups.

Urbanisation and literacy

We have seen that the Asian nations are ageing and developing at different rates, bringing about different rates of social change. Within each country, other factors such as degree and rate of urbanisation and improvements to literacy will also affect how they deal with their ageing populations.

Proportions of elderly in mega-cities often differ from those in the whole population or even in smaller cities. For example, Shanghai is relatively older than China's overall population, whereas Sendai is younger than the overall Japanese population. Sex ratios also vary between urban and rural areas. These are important considerations for targeting Australian promotional efforts. Less urbanised areas may be expected to respond more slowly to development and social change, regardless of their rate of ageing.

An aged population accustomed to high-density, high-rise apartment living has different expectations than villagers do. One Australian design for a nursing home in Singapore came temporarily unstuck over its plans for protected garden space.[8] The Australian consultants wanted it and tried to convince the local entrepreneur that it was necessary. Eventually, it became apparent that 'garden' was an alien concept for these urban elderly. What they wanted was a veranda to protect them from the heat and let them watch passers-by.

Improvements to literacy for women have long been associated with decreases in birth rates and childhood mortality. Literacy rates also feature in changing patterns of development, with less literate areas less responsive to changing circumstances. In China, for example, women's literacy rates are much lower than they are for men. For ages 50–59 years 33 per cent of women are literate compared to 72 per cent for men. For women 60+ the rates drop to 11 per cent, which indicates potential barriers to introducing new ideas about aged care services. Responding to the needs of rapidly ageing societies requires patience and understanding about the changes that older people have experienced over their lifetime.

Ageing accompanied by rapid development accentuates differences between younger and older women, increases generational conflict and complicates service delivery. As the feminist wave spreads, organised demands for education and health care are likely to rock patriarchal structures. Countries that fail to recognise the extra burdens that development places on women as both carers and workers may find they have unwittingly fermented feminine rebellion.

Political and economic context

Governments in the Asian region vary from military dictatorships to democracies tending towards openness. Most are considerably more volatile than those of Australia, which makes policy formulation less predictable. Official approaches to their ageing population varies from 'it's not an issue' to wanting to demonstrate that their services are world-class. Most have no tradition of public funding for aged care services, and the amount of government money available to alleviate the pressures of an ageing society varies greatly.

Some of the issues that will face governments are highly predictable. Developing countries will encounter an industrial relations aspect of providing aged care that is humane for both carers and staff. In some of them, 5-day 12-hour shifts are not considered unreasonable and the attitude that 'They are workers, and we will work them' is common. Considerations of quality of care are considered luxurious or indulgent. Other issues can be expected to arise from a clash with traditional values.

In some developing countries, many fear that if women move away from traditional roles as carers for the aged, social breakdown will occur. In some cases religious pressures are great enough to cause political stonewalling, which delays social adaptation.

In developing countries the medical profession is often strongly opposed to government interference in their domain, even when the organisation and delivery of services is obviously no longer appropriate to demographic changes. This echoes a struggle that took place in Australia over the last few decades (see Chapter 5), and is still occurring in some areas of aged care. On the positive side, by lobbying for better services to the elderly, and better conditions, wages and training for carers, the medical profession in these countries can make the transition to an aged society smoother by taking the initiative, as agents for change, when escalating costs force hard decisions on governments.

Health implications

Meeting the health care needs of the elderly is not a top priority for rapidly developing countries. When funds are available to expand health services, immediate concerns such as infant mortality and maintaining a healthy workforce tend to dominate planning. Despite the funding of health projects by groups like the World Bank,[9] developing countries still find it hard to finance improvements to health care. The preference for private sector funds for developments, along with the dominance of the medical profession, can create future problems with cost control and the choice of appropriate services. Malaysia, for example, is pursuing private sector health care funding at some pace in a shift away from its British style of public health system. Similarly, Thailand constructed 6500 new private hospital beds in 1995. It remains to be seen whether or not this has laid the foundations for American-style high-cost health care.

Over-reliance on private sector funding has implications for equity and social justice, while increased national wealth may make other solutions feasible. Some Australian companies are currently exploiting opportunities to develop multi-purpose facilities including facilities for the elderly. The longer-term issue will be the need to reorient the health system to the rapidly growing needs of the aged.

Good planning for these rapidly emerging health needs has to be based on solid research, and little is currently known about Asia's future health needs. Major differences in health patterns for its aged people may emerge. Women's needs are likely to be overlooked by a male-dominated and authoritarian medical system, highlighting yet another area in which Australian experience can be useful.

For example, women in the USA and Australia have expressed their dissatisfaction with the responsiveness of the health system in three areas not typically raised by men:

- violence and abuse as a health issue;
- mental health as a priority; and
- communication with doctors as a problem.

What issues will Asian women raise, if they are asked? This question is not merely rhetorical. Health care funding can always be assumed to be scarce, so careful targeting and communication planning is essential. It is also still to be determined what extra costs will be borne in old age by victims of arduous child labour and childhood prostitution in rapidly developing countries in Asia.

The AIDS epidemic is already starting to distort the demographics and health budget of some Asian nations, in a way not paralleled in Australia. One of Australia's great success stories is our early and sensible approach to AIDS education. Over the last few years, the number of cases of AIDS and HIV positive has stabilised. Australian experts offered assistance with AIDS prevention to Asian countries, notably Thailand and India, in the early stages of the epidemic. However, government commitment and money was too little too late.

Australian aged care expertise is also respected by Asian countries. In the new area of geriatrics and aged care we may find a more receptive audience because governments have a little longer to act and the aged are culturally valued. As argued in Chapter 4, an ageing society needs to reorient its health system towards preventing and alleviating disability instead of taking expensive and sometimes heroic measures to prevent death. Some of the poorer countries may find this adjustment easier, as the means for hi-tech intervention just won't be affordable.

Providing adequate nursing staff and changing people's attitudes to dementia will present a major challenge. In many developing areas, training for nurses is inferior by Australian standards, and Philippina nurses are often imported to alleviate staff shortages. 'We started our training program with hand washing and went on from there,' said one consultant about the skills base of nursing home staff at one south-east Asian facility.[10]

What can we offer?

In contrast to Asian countries, Australia has consistently expected its government to have a major hand in providing for its aged citizens. The public sector has never supplanted family care, but has been there to complement and relieve the family. This public involvement has grown, as more women in the workforce and an ageing society have increased the burdens on family and volunteer carers. The development of aged care services in Australia may illustrate another aspect of cultural convergence, if Asian countries repeat our history in this aspect. Australia has indeed come a long way from the harsh attitudes that characterised treatments of the aged early in this century.

Over several decades, we have also developed experience in research and planning for aged care, as well as the bricks and mortar of design and funding. We now have particular expertise in home and community services, nursing homes, and housing for the aged. This expertise has developed in a philosophical framework that is culturally very different to that of our Asian neighbours. However, Asia is changing culturally as it matures. Our services will be most appreciated if the planners have enough vision to foresee change and provide for it flexibly. There's no point in designing services or buildings that will be obsolete or redundant in a short time.

For example, an Australian architect had a difficult time convincing his Japanese client that toilets placed along outside walls, with natural light and ventilation, were necessary for hygiene and also just for pleasantness. He saw this as important, because, he said, 'We're designing to cover our future, recognising the potential for growth and change'.

Australia's medical insurance and aged care systems are recognised around the world for their equity and efficiency. Part of their strength is a continuing scrutiny of systems and openness to further reform. If our Asian neighbours decide to 'bite the bullet' and consider greater government support for aged care, they may well turn to us for guidance. Both in our financial accountability systems and our outcome-oriented standards of care (as outlined in Chapter 5), Australia illustrates what government involvement in aged care can achieve. If true respect for the dignity and well-being of the elderly is the goal, we have the products to achieve it.

Servicing the client

Many of the cultural differences present obstacles from both sides. For example, Australians may come up with standards of design or function that don't interest their Asian clients, even though the clients want to measure up to established standards. Finding the best compromise involves negotiations that are partly cultural and partly financial. Often a joint venture is the best solution, because both sides have commitment and understanding. The overseas partner is well placed to deal with the authorities at that end and provide feedback on local needs.

Starting from square one

Australian expertise in aged care research, planning and implementation is long-standing, and of a high quality. Because this is largely government-funded, our bureaucrats and the academics who assist them have much to contribute at the government level. In the workplace, aged care needs have to be recognised as part of other family responsibilities. This is also an area in which the Australian government has cut a bold path, as part of our obligations as signatory to International Labour Organisation Convention 156 on Workers with Family Responsibilities. We are developing much more family-friendly workplaces through such measures as flexible working hours and special leave provisions. Already, elder care responsibilities are becoming an issue for such policies in Australian workplaces. Here, too, competitive Asian economies may benefit from our experience. Such adjustments for families with ageing relatives may prove more cost-effective than the loss of highly skilled personnel.

At the bricks and mortar level, our architects and engineers are already designing and building hospitals and other health care facilities. At the human resources level, our health professionals, nursing schools and technical colleges are already involved in both 'training the trainers' and setting up service delivery programs.

Residential care

Old people's homes are an important option for public services that assist not only older people but also their families. Best practice, family-style homes are rare throughout the developing world, as they were in developed countries like Australia ten or more years ago, but they are developing fast. Australian firms are already developing such facilities in Japan and Singapore. Here Australia has a great opportunity to contribute hard-won intellectual capital. Our model is considered advanced because it is 'upstream from a community model' rather than 'downstream from a medical model'. Countries like Japan are still caught up in the medical model, and resist paying for 'soft matter' in the form of philosophies of care and their application. The social pressures of rapid ageing are already leading to experiments with different structures, particularly in Japan.

Part of the intellectual capital we offer consists of our clearly stated standards for aged care in nursing homes and hostels. Because these are defined by outcomes rather than inputs, they are adaptable for other circumstances. The standards themselves are not immutable, but are based on respect and dignity for the individual. No-one ageing now in Australia would regard these as luxuries.

Home services

This option has been successful in Australia, both economically and socially. We accept the need for publicly funded services to the aged, in their homes. Such services are developing rapidly in wealthy countries but are less common in developing countries. Cultural differences, as we have seen, make this option less acceptable at the present in Asia, and public funding is less likely.

Demographics may override cultural resistance. In Japan in the 1990s one out of 15 women is expected to care for senile or bedridden elderly, whereas by 2025 that ratio is expected to be one in two.[11] The family/traditional support strategy for care is no longer tenable on its own.

The ambitious Japanese 10-year 'Gold Plan'[12] aims to develop home-delivered services to deal with the very rapid growth in numbers of very old. This development confronts several barriers, including the need to increase taxes to pay for the new services, the opposition of the medical profession to services that they do not control, and Japan's lack of a tradition of public welfare.

Day care and multi-purpose centres

Another alternative is centres outside the home which provide a wide range of therapy services, with an emphasis on rehabilitation. In Australia, these are important in preventing inappropriate admissions to nursing homes. In rural areas, multi-purpose centres provide the flexibility to meet the diverse age care needs of a smaller population. As these services tend to follow medical models, Asian countries may find them more acceptable than unrelated carers coming to the home.

Training plus tourism

Services and skills require training, and some Australian aged care providers are already offering to overseas groups packages that combine recreation with first-hand experience of how an efficient nursing home works. One respected provider of integrated services, based in Ballarat, Victoria, has developed for visiting Japanese aged care workers flexible training packages that can include facility management, financial administration, and service planning. Visits to tourist locations round out the all-in-one-fee package.

Such an approach offers spin-offs for other local industries. The Ballarat example brought in the local TAFE to develop the service, on a commission basis. Along the way, local hotels and restaurants learned a lot about catering to Japanese needs, several interpreters found employment, and the owner of the Australian aged care facility has joined a new age experts network group to help keep up to date on export developments and to improve communications. An important feature of this training package is its emphasis on caring for the rights and needs of the nursing home residents. Seeking permission before bringing strangers into their home, and paying attention to other people's reactions and sensitivities has helped to make the program a success.

International students and consultancies

Active recruiting overseas has increased the numbers of students enrolling in Australian university courses, many of them from rapidly ageing Asian nations. This, in turn, leads to another benefit, as these students often go on to high level positions in their governments and provide good contacts for Australian expertise. Exposure to Australia's high standards of aged care sometimes prompts Asian countries to set up consultancy opportunities for our gerontologists. Several are now providing Total Quality Management packages, from design and fittings to staffing and financial administration, for nursing homes in Asia.

Current activity in exporting aged care

Government interest in this area dates from at least 1991, when the Department of Human Services and Health advertised a consultancy to investigate the export opportunities that an ageing Asia might offer Australia. The issue here is not whether we export but how we coordinate and expand the exports. At the moment it is not a large market, but the rapidly increasing numbers of elderly with rising per capita income in Asian countries, indicate that it is ripe for further development. As an analogy, who would have seriously thought 10 years ago that Australian tertiary education would become a significant export industry, worth 1.5 billion dollars in 1994? There is similar potential for aged care. The Australian interest involves a humanitarian concern and the addition of profit to a sector that we normally think of as entirely dependent on government funding. Exports can improve Australia's resources for providing high-quality services to its own population in an environment where other aged care funding sources are tightly constrained.

Australia needs to develop networks of exporters and experts to promote the development of high-quality exports. Public sector officials need to become more knowledgeable about Asia through education and experience in regional activities. The Australian involvement in exporting aged care expertise has the potential to match the achievements in exporting Australian education services. The emerging Australian Aged Care Exporters (AACE) Network will be a select group of experienced exporters who will develop high-quality exports.

Conclusion

Many questions confront Australians when it comes to engaging in this 'greenfield' area. What should be the extent and nature of public sector involvement in the industry? How should networks of exporters and experts be organised and resourced? What should exporters charge for these services? We are beginning to make ground on these issues. It is clear that the government's role will be to establish the process of exporting, remove the barriers and make the government-level contacts. Exporters will themselves be responsible for export activities.

These issues are discussed in the consultancy Report on Exporting Aged Care Services[13] and priorities for action have been set out. If we take the issue of which countries take priority for export, the Report nominated Japan at the top and placed Indonesia well down the list. However, our market research[14] indicates Indonesia as the country that people most wanted to learn about. Was the Export Report wrong or short-sighted? The more recent Booz-Allen and Hamilton[15] report on health exports to Indonesia devotes a short chapter to aged care. It starts by stating: 'Today aged care is not a current priority in Indonesia', continues with 'even by the year 2010 aged care is unlikely to be a priority', and concludes by saying 'potential opportunities in the near-term are few and small'. Despite the observations of Booz-Allen and Hamilton there may be skilful people who can find a niche in Indonesia. The point is that it is not good strategy for new players to start in such a market when higher priority needs exist elsewhere. Any activities in Indonesia will depend on private companies or government Foreign Aid money.

What we need is further information and discussion on these issues. This assumes a developing interest by public and private sector participants in Australia's aged care. Australians need an efficient system that can develop their knowledge about ageing in Asia. The role of the public sector as a central point for information and for the coordination of developments is vital.

Networks of academic and applied experts and exporters must be developed and maintained. Since they do not yet communicate with one another there is a lack of synergy in the work of both parties. The primary goal of this networking is more to do with international exchange than profit. Aligning our ageing policies and expertise with Asian experience will give us new points of comparison and new ideas. It will also prompt us to discover and maintain international best practice in aged care services. In many situations the motive for international exchange will be to help rather than to earn income. People may do this out of altruism or funded by a foreign government aid agency. On the other hand we should not naively sell ourselves short to sharp overseas entrepreneurs.

Countries with organised marketing have generally done better than those whose exporters do not pool their efforts and who are made to compete against one another for contracts. In terms of the public sector we should be looking to a future where senior staff are much better informed about Asia through education and exposure to regional meetings. As interest in practical skills increases in Asia, a program of exchanges will be required to develop public sector experts' sensitivity to the needs and practices of top priority Asian countries. In the immediate future those countries are Japan and the Chinese expatriate communities in Singapore, Hong Kong, Taiwan and throughout the Asia Pacific region. This will expand to cover most of the rapidly developing countries of north-east and south-east Asia in the near future. As the Commonwealth report cited early in the chapter optimistically observes: 'there appears to be almost unlimited potential for Australia to participate in the rapidly developing Asian aged care market'.

Notes

1 Commonwealth Dept of Human Services and Health 1994, *Exporting Australia's Aged Care Services to Asia*, AGPS, Canberra.

2 McCallum, J. 1995, 'Exporting aged care services to Asia: Regional trends and Australian responses'. In J. McCallum (ed.), *Export of Aged Care Services Training*, National Centre for Epidemiology and Population Health, Canberra.

3 McCallum, J. and Osteria, T. 1991, *Evaluation of the UNFPA-Supported Project 'Creation of Awareness on Aging for Policy Making Purposes in the Asian Region'*, Japanese Ministry of Foreign Affairs and UNFPA, Tokyo.

4 Kinsella, K. 1988, *Aging in the Third World*, US Bureau of the Census, International Population Reports Series P–95, No. 79, Washington.

5 Kinsella, K. and Taeuber, C.M. 1993, *An Aging World II*, US Bureau of the Census, International Population Reports Series P–95, 92–3, Washington.

6 McCallum and Osteria, *Evaluation of the UNFPA-Supported Project*.

7 Myers, G. 1992, 'Demographic Aging and Family Support for Older Persons'. In H.L. Kendig, Hashimoto, A. and Coppard, L.C. (eds) *Family Support for the Elderly: The International Experience*, Oxford University Press, Tokyo, pp. 31–68.

8 McCallum, 'Exporting aged care services to Asia'.

9 World Bank 1993, *Investing in Health*, World Bank Development Report 1993, Oxford University Press, New York.

10 McCallum, 'Exporting aged care services to Asia'.

11 Ogawa, N. 1993, *An Analysis of Medical Issues of a Society with Extremely Low Birth Rates—Based on the Integrated Model*, Nihon University Population Research Institute, Tokyo.

12 Japanese Ministry of Health and Welfare 1990, *Ten Year Strategy to Promote Healthcare and Welfare for the Aged*, Ministry of Health and Welfare, Tokyo.

13 See Note 1.

14 McCallum, Exporting aged care services to Asia'.

15 Booz-Allen and Hamilton Australia Ltd 1995, *Maximising Australia's Health Industry Export Potential to Indonesia*, Report commissioned by DHSH, DIST, DEET, Market Australia and Austrade.

8

The new aged confront the third millennium

A good and decent life in old age has a natural appeal, as does the image of a healthy laughing child. But neither happens automatically through the 'nature of things'. As we have seen, harsh attitudes towards the elderly were common in early Australia and problems persist even now. Clearly, most older people can have a rewarding and satisfying old age, despite their greater physical and social vulnerability. The outcome depends on both the individual and the social context. Citizenship and lifelong contributions give them a claim to public support, but this has to be widely recognised—by the elderly as well as by others. This recognition is evolving, as our actions today help to construct citizenship for tomorrow's elderly.

Throughout this book, we have tried to 'deconstruct' the political and economic structures that inhibit the full social participation of the elderly. Although we have many excellent policies, others are not so benign and will have to be changed or replaced to suit our ageing population. Stereotypes and maladaptive structures persist, and make it difficult for older people to create a positive identity. Older people need not only the material means but also the knowledge and encouragement to live a 'good' life in their later years. In order to meet the challenge of ageing in an increasingly individualistic society, we must first reaffirm our collective social obligations. There are many different points of view on this issue in our post-modern culture.

The concept of citizenship has evolved in Western societies to include more rights and responsibilities for individuals. Some examples of this are the right to an adequate income in old age, established at the beginning of this century, and the access to humane residential and

> If the universe has not been constructed in accordance with any plan, it has no meaning to be discovered. There is no value inherent in it, independently of the existence of sentient beings who prefer some states of affairs to others. Ethics is not part of the structure of the universe, in the way that atoms are.
>
> . . . no amount of reflection will show a commitment to an ethical life to be trivial or pointless. This is probably the most important claim in this book, but also the most contentious.
>
> Peter Singer 1993, How Are We to Live?
Ethics in an age of self-interest, Text
Publishing, Sydney, pp. 188, 218.

community care instigated progressively after World War II. Australia has concentrated on equal treatment, flat-rate pensions and access to nursing homes independent of consumers' means. Policies are now changing, so that contributions differ according to access, for example in superannuation and hostel care. Diversity and individual treatment are the imperatives of post-modern societies. We saw in the last chapter how Australia's enlightened expertise in aged care is greatly sought after. We also had a glimpse of what can happen when long-accepted entitlements are subordinated to private greed, with public blessing.

Administratively, the recognition of individual differences and diversity introduces an expensive complexity to 'post-modern' government policies. While the technology for dealing with the massive amounts of data which run today's governmental systems has expanded exponentially, so has the public's demand for access to information. The generation working now is the first to be flooded with information, and to grasp its potential to help them control their lives.

The halcyon days of generous welfare support are at an end, as governments find that the demands upon them exceed their capacity to raise revenue. In addition, the basic safety net levels of income and of services that worked in the past won't seem generous or even adequate to the workers approaching old age now. The elderly of today are 'the lucky generation' who have experienced sustained economic and employment growth. The employment opportunities benefited women only indirectly since they were mostly marginal in or excluded from the workforce. Today's elderly have benefited from the expansion of public health and welfare.

The good news for the baby boomers is that they are riding the crest of a wave that has given their generation in developed countries the highest material standard of living the world has ever known. This is why claims of intergenerational inequity are misplaced. We owe a debt to the older generation who created this growth and few begrudge them decent treatment in old age. Along with longevity, this affluence has brought freedom, tolerance, and information. There is greater access to the legal, medical, social and consumer structures and data that form the basis of policy formation and program delivery.

Tomorrow's elderly will need all the information they can get, just to manage and make sense of the constant change around them. The former, happy coincidence of contingencies that produced sustained economic growth after World War II is now out of alignment and Australia's future is caught up in the uncertainties of the international marketplace. Another 25 years of sustained growth are unlikely after the next recession. In any case, the old type of growth would be undesirable. We are discovering first-hand that growth has limits, that the planet itself is vulnerable, and that we have an obligation to leave adequate resources for following generations.

Today's elderly are pursuing the right to participate in all aspects of public decision-making. We expect this trend to accelerate with tomorrow's aged, and have indicated how it will serve both social and economic goals. Already, older people are redefining citizenship, and its minimal parameters. For example, in the 19th century the arbitrated wage took into account the cost of a daily newspaper, considered a social necessity at the time.[1] Will future costs of citizenship include optical fibre access to global information networks?

In this final chapter we outline some of the structural inadequacies that restrict the full citizenship of older people, and where further developments are likely to occur. Euthanasia is perhaps the most emotive issue for debate over rights. The right to die is most challenging to the benevolent paternalism with which we treat older people.

The other aspect of rights is, of course, responsibilities. In the past, the aged were often considered useless. Recent generations have established that they can and do contribute in many ways. Examples such as SeniorNet[2] run by an 80-year-old in Queensland, show how the aged can still contribute to social capital, if favourable structures are put in place. The aged are a valuable resource for the future. This is a sign of recognition, not exploitation.

We place particular emphasis on the rapid development of information technology for research, access and activism. This access to information is important not only in caring for the current elderly but also to ensure equity for the future. In health, consumerism, obstacles to late-life employment, housing, politics and education, today's elderly have started down new avenues. We predict that tomorrow's aged will turn these into highways as they seek enrichment and enhancement in their golden years. Technology's promise to the aged is alluring.[3] However, as healthy retirement inevitably gives way to greater dependency, we must gracefully acknowledge this and provide the care that technology cannot give.

Health and care rights

In Chapter 5 we gave some examples of older people's health care being brutally inconsiderate and inappropriate, as well as wasteful of health care dollars. The key issue was that the wishes of older people were not being respected, in fact they were rarely spoken to when things went awry. The remedy includes changing the communication training for professional health workers, raising general awareness about these problems, and providing open and accountable information to all groups with an interest in this area.

Generally, older people and those most intimately involved with their care are best placed to comment on the services involved. The new wave of policy formulation for the aged described in Chapter 2 asks for and takes account of people's stated needs. This should lead to better outcomes all round, especially if it is used in conjunction with the growing trend of 'evidence-based medicine'.

Evidence-based medicine

One might ask, with some alarm, how there could be any other kind of medicine. Isn't medicine a science? Unfortunately, doctors are only human and medicine is as much an art as a science. Their function is constrained by the limited evidence that they are aware of, as well as by the limited vision that they derive from their personal and social context. In a world awash with information, this is no longer enough to produce the best outcomes for patients. Good science tends to be based on randomised controlled trials (RCTs), which have safeguards to prevent observer bias in the results. Surprisingly, not all medical research is conducted in this rigorous way. And much good research is written up in foreign languages or in obscure journals. The average practising doctor has no way of keeping up with the latest research, and his or her skills can deteriorate after medical training.

In 1972 the British doctor Archie Cochrane wrote a pathbreaking book *Effectiveness and Efficiency: Random Reflections on Health Services* in which he drew attention to the collective ignorance about the effects of health care and to the fact that reliable reviews of evidence were not readily available to those who make decisions about health care—professionals and consumers. In 1979 in a critical review of the medical profession he wrote: 'It is surely a great criticism of our profession that we have not organised a critical summary, by specialty or subspecialty, adapted periodically, of all relevant randomised controlled trials.'

Archie Cochrane lived long enough to see the systematic review of RCTs of care during pregnancy and childbirth released in 1987, the year before he died. He referred to this as a 'real milestone in the history of randomised trials and in the evaluation of care' and recommended the method to other specialty areas. In his last year of life he was pleased to discover a well designed randomised trial that demonstrated how different ways of providing supportive care for the dying and their families variously affected their quality of life.

The Australian Cochrane Centre, opened in 1995 in Adelaide, and based on the Centre for Evidence-Based Medicine at Oxford University, is changing all this. A team there is working to sift through the masses of research, highlighting the work based on good RCTs, and making it available via the Cochrane database of systematic reviews. The task is huge, so they are going about it systematically, taking on each disease and condition as groups around the world volunteer to make systematic reviews. An example of the success of this approach was the abandonment of certain drugs to control erratic heartbeat, after an analysis of RCTs revealed that they actually decreased chances of survival.

The Cochrane Database of Systematic Reviews is being published on computer discs, CD ROM and the Internet. So if you see your doctor referring to a computer before deciding on treatment, it could be that some of the world's best information is at his or her fingertips. Equally important, it will become easier for doctors and health care consumers to discuss treatment options from a mutually informed perspective.

Only a few collaborations deal specifically with ageing issues but we can expect these topics to grow rapidly as the legacy of Archie Cochrane spreads. Older people's access to this rich resource is a difficult issue, as retired people have been identified as among the least likely to own a personal computer. However, as current workers enter old age this type of collaborative decision-making may become the norm. An undue reliance on formal, 'scientific' investigations of the effects of care was never Cochrane's idea. The non-specific effects of care and love are often major determinants of health care outcomes. However, while well designed evaluations of the effects of care are not sufficient for improving health care decisions, they remain essential for making these decisions better informed.

Whose informed consent?

However much information is made available to consumers there will still be a disparity of information between doctors and patients. This can easily become a power gap, particularly if the patient is elderly or unquestioning. The doctor's responsibility to inform patients about the effects of any intervention has both an ethical and a defensive aspect. Many malpractice suits arise over lack of 'informed consent', where the patient claims they did not have all aspects of treatment explained to them before they agreed to it. It is generally left to the doctor's judgement to decide how much to tell a patient, how much they seem capable of grasping, to what extent they can or should have a say in determining their own treatment, and at what point to call in another relative to assist in the decision.

This obligation also applies to all situations regardless of the threat of litigation, including the prescription of pharmaceuticals, the ordering of diagnostic tests and other therapies. Such situations may arise more frequently with older patients, who often suffer multiple conditions and are given multiple medications unnecessarily. There is a tendency to treat them as lesser persons who need not be informed because they are incapable of dealing with the information. On the other hand, it is often the case that the doctor is not fully informed about the side effects and complications of a particular treatment. How then can the patient hope to make a wise decision? And what rights do relatives and loved ones have, considering the responsibilities they have?

For controversial alternative treatments, there is room for much more truly scientific assessment. Sir William Keys,[4] formerly national president of the RSL, claims that his prostate cancer has been cured by a combination of western medicine, Chinese herbal medicine and his own positive mental attitude and meditation. He points out that Chinese medicine has been developed by trial and error over centuries. The medical profession is slowly starting to consider, after much resistance, a whole range of therapies once thought 'loopy'. There is also an imperative that these alternatives be as safe and as beneficial as conventional treatments. As the population ages and the incidence of degenerative diseases increases, self-experimentation is bound to come up with a few surprises. These must be rigorously examined on their merits. For example, the role of antioxidants such as vitamin C and E are now acknowledged, as is the harmful cumulative effect of agricultural chemicals. A key problem is how to prise rebates for more appropriate services from the hands of the medical profession. Apart from the well-off, future generations of elderly are not likely to be able to afford the luxury of private, alternative treatments.

Death with dignity—the last 'rights'?

In Greek mythology Charon was the ferryman who took passengers across the River Styx, the divide between the living and the dead. Medical technology and drugs now tend to place doctors in the position of Charon. They are often pressured into making life and death decisions about patients who are moribund or whose quality of life is severely diminished. While we all know stories about elderly people who 'just let go' and slipped away, many others have suffered horribly for much too long.

The Hippocratic oath requires doctors to 'do no harm'. Hastening or causing death would seem to violate these revered principles. Of course, many treatments cause short-term harm for long-term good, including chemotherapy and even cosmetic treatment. The 'triage' system of priority-setting has been a common feature of wartime medical care (i.e. dividing patients into three categories: those requiring immediate attention, those whose medical treatment can be delayed, and those whom treatment will not save), however deliberately limiting medical care in an affluent peacetime setting is not considered acceptable. The profusion of choice at both ends of life has led to confusion. Although it is hard to argue that the decision on when to end life should be taken from the dying, opponents to euthanasia claim that similar 'watertight' legislation has been abused overseas, and will undoubtedly lead to non-consensual deaths here.

Because it involves deliberately causing death, the concept of euthanasia is much more difficult than that of simply withholding treatment. In between lies palliative care which seeks to ease the path to a 'natural death'. One difficulty is that such care may not be adequate, either emotionally or medically. Patients caught in the inadvertent brutality of helplessness and pain may feel that suicide or euthanasia are their only alternatives. In our rushed society, some even want to hasten death, rather than allowing it to occur in its own time and space, cushioned and guided by loved ones.

Legislation passed in the Northern Territory in mid 1995 has given Australia international prominence on this issue by making deliberate death legal under tightly controlled conditions. Other states and territories are expected to follow suit, although similar legislation was rejected in South Australia. 'Living wills' or advanced notices which state under what conditions certain kinds of care or treatments are to be withheld, should the person be incapable of deciding, can provide a form of insurance against the unnecessary and unwelcome prolongment of life. These could cover many cases, but not the common situation where the patient is quite lucid, is not on life support equipment, but is in horrible distress or pain with no relief possible.

Another common situation occurs when the patient is demented, but not in danger of death. In such a case euthanasia is out of the question, even though quality and dignity of life may be vastly diminished. This highly emotive area already has its lobby groups, such as the Dying with Dignity Action Group, who recommends legalising Living Wills and registering them on a national database. Public pressure and the desire of the baby boomers to record their wishes and exercise control in this final aspect of their lives may accelerate the debate rapidly over the next few decades. The entire 'end of life' web of care and support has to be humane enough to respond to suffering by concentrating on people rather than medicine.

Discrimination

Earlier this century, people were considered elderly at much younger ages than they are today, partly because of shorter life expectancies. Blatant assumptions about the elderly being useless and pathetic were often seen in the newspapers, and were little questioned. The wage earners' welfare state gave its older members pensions in lieu of work participation.

Concepts of citizenship, recognition of diversity and feminism are just some of the social changes that have altered perceptions since those days of mindless stereotyping. Today, many conflicts over 'ageism' involve economic issues, notably employment. Australia is signatory to International Labor Organisation Covenant 111, concerning discrimination in employment and occupation. This is incorporated in federal law in the

Human Rights and Equal Opportunity Commission Act. However, complaints can be pursued all the way to the High Court for resolution. It can be time-consuming and expensive, and the outcome is uncertain. Complaints are usually resolved by conciliation. Most States and Territories have specific discrimination legislation covering the aged, as part of their broader anti-discrimination provisions. They often back this up with guidelines and information brochures for employers.

Despite legislative protection, the numbers of those retiring before 65 are increasing, not all voluntarily. Many others want or need to remain in the workforce, perhaps past 65. They will probably find this increasingly difficult, as workers over 45 are often considered less desirable. As in the United States, there are many structural rigidities set up to discourage the employment of older workers. For example, under the Superannuation Industry Supervision (SIS) Act 1993 contributions cannot be made to a super scheme once the contributing employee turns 65. New technologies are already making it easier to work from home, and extend working lives considerably. Growing inequality in job distribution, and greater reliance on earning for retirement income will catch many workers between a rock and a hard place.

Meanwhile, several States and the Commonwealth Public Service are moving to lift the compulsory retirement age of 65. For those with secure job tenure, this could be a lifeline to an adequate livelihood. Many others, particularly those with adequate superannuation, prefer early retirement, usually in their pursuit of a better quality of life. Not surprisingly, the kinds of adaptation necessary to retain older employees are similar to those found successful in assisting workers with young children: flexible working hours, training and promotional opportunities, adaptive technology, recognition of caring responsibilities, part-time work and phased retirement. As the wave of ageing crests, the focus of government compliance with ILO 156 on Workers with Family Responsibilities is likely to shift somewhat towards elder care responsibilities. Since access to family care is a critical variable in keeping the frail and disabled elderly out of residential care, the availability of carers has important ramifications.

Consumer rights and obligations

The assembling and sharing of electronic information about consumer rights and responsibilities will probably grow at least as rapidly as the information superhighway. The Australian Federation of Consumer Organisations operates from a firm base and is well aware of the problems older consumers face. Other community groups, such as the Council on the Aged, ACOSS, the Australian Pensioners and Superannuants Federation, and the Older Women's Network keep a watching brief, conduct research and make submissions to governments on areas of interest to the elderly.

Superannuation is a particularly troublesome area for the elderly, and obtaining accurate information is often the greatest hurdle. An independent Superannuation Complaints Tribunal has been set up by the Commonwealth government to resolve some complaints concerning super, and the provision of information is an important obligation of funds regulated by the Superannuation Industry Supervision Act.

The public right to know and Freedom of Information legislation

The information technology explosion will make it easier for governments to formulate and evaluate policies and programs, by opening up the process to interested individuals and organisations. Those who do not grasp this opportunity will find themselves under fire to reveal their data. Pricing and other aspects of Freedom of Information legislation are crucial to this move towards 'open systems'.

Pricing and content policies on the Internet are currently being debated, as more information goes up daily through networks open to the public. One list of government-initiated multi-media and electronic access projects was over 30 pages long.[5] The Internet offers savings here on paper, postage, and phone staff. It is also vital, in the interests of efficiency and full citizenship, to take full advantage of these new technologies. This means systems must be interactive, and used creatively for policy formulation, implementation and modification. The information should be accessible to all interested parties, without censorship. This is a tall bill, but initiatives such as the Community Information Network in the Department of Social Security have great potential.[6]

The Federal Office of Government Information and Advertising sets out guidelines for Australian Government Information Activities.[7] These specify that any group which is 'disadvantaged through low income, poor education, inadequate knowledge of English, physical handicap, geographical isolation or any other reason' is 'information poor', and that departments must give special attention to these groups when preparing their information programs. Mention is made of young people, the rural community, those for whom English is not a convenient language in which to receive information, women, ethnic communities, and Aboriginal and Torres Strait Islander communities.

These guidelines stipulate that at least 7.5 per cent of the campaign budget allocated to newspaper advertising must be devoted to non-English language media. The aged population is not mentioned specifically as a disadvantaged group, perhaps because they are too disparate and varied. *Age Pension News*, a large print publication from the Department of Social Security, is one example of government information produced for the elderly.

Housing and urban design

The ageing of the population poses many challenges for our cities. It is no coincidence that many aspects of planning towns and housing for an ageing society overlap with good environmental practice. The elderly can be seen as part of the 'social capital' which must be conserved if we are to have social, as well as environmental sustainability.

In practical terms, this means that creating 'ghettos' for the aged is counter-productive. Keeping the streets safe and accessible for the aged and for their grandchildren creates a seamless neighbourhood. Much work has been done on crime prevention, and on planning transport and housing for multi-generational use. Forms of co-housing, based on European models, are emerging in Australia. These involve the limited pooling of resources in small-scale (and therefore manageable) ventures among, perhaps, a group of 8–10 families so that they have separate homes but share a communal space and some activities. It is easy to see how the elderly could be incorporated in such an arrangement, which would bear some resemblance to rural Asian multi-generational compounds. What can no longer be adequately provided by a single, much diminished family unit is partially replaced by the group arrangement.

A strategy paper prepared by the Australian Urban and Regional Development Review[8] recommends change to housing stock to give older people more choice. There are certainly possibilities here for moving away from the institutional aspect of retirement housing in favour of joint ventures that will be economical, efficient, and help to form bonds of care and assistance.

The redundancy of modern buildings is a problem that often affects the elderly. As with our export efforts to Asia, we need to ensure that we are designing for a future of diversity and flexibility. The waste of materials when buildings become redundant, as well as unnecessary energy use, maintenance and repairs are all growing concerns for environmental architects.[9] Such housing costs are often a major drain on older people's resources. A more commonsense approach to durability could also include designing opportunities for greater resource sharing and for encouraging social interdependency, to replace the extreme and expensive forms of individual autonomy we relish in today's suburbs.

Housing and the interactions it fosters are vital, but design for an ageing society will reach much further. Not all, or even most elderly will be disabled, but total numbers will be greater than today. Many will also fall into a grey zone of arthritis or impaired vision or hearing, of being frustrated by hard-to-read instrument displays in their cars. Teller machines, computer terminals, bottles, labels, handrails, clothing—these are just some of the areas that will have to be adjusted to the needs of the aged. Clearly, there is enormous market potential here, and enormous scope for conflict if expectations are not met. Already seminars are being offered on 'Marketing to the over 50's'.[10]

Neither abuse nor ignore

Even those once considered most vulnerable and least able to speak out—the residents of nursing homes and hostels—now have a voice. As well as a charter of rights, these people now have advocacy services and procedures for protest against ill treatment. These, unfortunately, have more to do with redress than with outcomes. The generally inferior power status of these residents raises the question of how realistic such rights are. Ultimately, if society is 'looking the other way', recognition of rights becomes a private matter of conscience, professionalism and judgement on the part of the carer.[11]

A similar situation applies in a non-institutional setting. Abuse of the aged in the home is an ugly area, and difficult because older people usually depend on their abusers. Police departments and welfare groups are working to find ways of dealing with this problem. Unfortunately, the elderly can't be fostered out as children can. Caring for the elderly is an often undervalued service, and many of the elderly are themselves carers. Burdens of care can create health risks for carers, and there is already great demand on home care and respite services. New approaches to urban design and service delivery which develop, rather than erode, social capital can offer solutions here.

Community values

The loss of social capital in Australian urban communities makes a serious impact on the aged, one that is less pronounced in rural communities except when they become depopulated. The loss is caused by the pervasive pragmatism of modern people, the effects of big government and big business, the complexities of immigration and the failures of policy design. Bush fire brigades are typical of what can be achieved by unpaid volunteers when the calculation of benefits and gains is replaced by community cooperation.

The loss of community leaves the elderly without traditional contacts and supports. They are forced into an impoverished social life which makes self-care and self-sufficiency more difficult. As a group, they have developed a fear of crime out of proportion to the real incidence of crime. In extreme situations, their very lives may be forfeited for lack of community. A prolonged heatwave in the United States led to the deaths of hundreds of people in mid 1995, a disproportionate number of them elderly, poor urban dwellers. Some had no-one to turn to for assistance, others were afraid to open their windows, others couldn't afford life-saving airconditioners. Australians beware!

Conclusion

These issues give an indication of how and where the current generation of aged and the future elderly will change the shape of society. Hopefully, their activism and demands will exert a positive influence on policy-makers and service delivery, and lead to efficient public outlays. It is also clear that there is an obligation on the aged to continue their participation, according to their inclinations and abilities, and to maintain an awareness of the generations that follow. No less is the obligation on younger groups to plan and provide. Sociobiologists studying both simulated and real populations have gone beyond the concept of 'selfish genes' to recognise that seemingly altruistic behaviour can be the most adaptive in the long term.

The light on the hill

We have a great objective—the light on the hill—which we aim to reach by working for the betterment of mankind not only here but anywhere we may give a helping hand.

J.B. Chifley, speech to NSW ALP conference, June 1949.

The famous 'light on the hill' phrase was a beacon for benign welfare policies for several decades. While working for the betterment of mankind may be an unquestionable goal, we can examine the concept of a 'helping hand' more critically. The statement was made when Australia was still a fully egalitarian society. Indeed, in the early 1970s the gap between the lowest and highest quintile of incomes could be bridged by an extra 9-hour per week part-time job. Employment was plentiful, compared with today. It was reasonable to offer 'a helping hand' to the less fortunate, and to assume that those who helped had not created the need for welfare in the first place.

Society's complexity has multiplied since then, and our population has nearly doubled. Australia is following the trend of other OECD countries towards inequality, and we have become increasingly dependent on overseas events for our economic health. Earlier forms of democracy, which seemed to work in a pre-media, pre-information age, no longer deliver to a disgruntled electorate. Logically, structures for participation must broaden, and feedback loops must be set up to pry open the many 'cans of worms' that twist and turn and lead to undesirable outcomes. Too many cracks in formerly impregnable fortresses of authority are appearing. The 'helping hand' is now required to offer power, not welfare. At stake is our sustainability.

The elements of a sustainable society are not mysterious. In a holistic paper on older age structures, environment and social change, a husband and wife team, Lincoln and Alice Day,[12] outline the pathways to a society that supports all groups. They emphasise the importance of both the built and natural environments in creating social cohesion, as well as the importance of establishing a more equal distribution of wealth. Certainly in terms of distribution of wealth, and especially in the last two decades, Australia moved further away from this ideal, and that failure undermines all other social goals. Several studies have demonstrated that the cycle of disadvantage is becoming more entrenched, that the wealthier sectors have better health, better education, better jobs, earlier and more affluent retirement. Their neighbourhoods have less crime, their children marry into higher socio-economic groups, and so it goes. Why does this matter so much, since, some might say, the poor will always be with us? It matters because the policy-makers are among the 'haves', and will never act to disadvantage themselves. This becomes crucial when issues such as public accountability, efficiency and true rationalism are taken into consideration. Greater inequity inevitably perpetuates self-serving attitudes and a determination to cling to power—that is the way of the world and of human nature. Australia has a long and noble history of caring for the underdog, of protecting the helpless and giving everyone 'a fair go'. This has been the great strength of our public policies, and it has developed over decades when we also valued our mateship and egalitarianism, despite a concurrent tendency to ageism, racism and sexism.

The generation now in their most productive and powerful years, those born in the period of recovery after World War II, stand at the cusp. If there is any chance that the world is more dangerously vulnerable, overcrowded and environmentally degraded than ever before, then we have just a little while to tilt the balance back towards stability. On the other hand, if our age is just another example of being born in 'interesting times', then we should cautiously proceed on the same path towards sustainability, equity and social cohesion. We owe it to ourselves, our parents, and our children.

As we move towards the 'hill' of ageing which the new aged represent, we will have to consciously reach past immediate costs and complexities to think and plan for the plateau of sustainability which lies beyond. Only if each of us embraces this view for the longer haul can we congratulate ourselves on having lived well.

Notes

1 Sawer, M. 1995, 'The Citizenship Debate', *The Australia Institute Newsletter*, No. 4, June.
2 SeniorNet is sponsored by Global Infolinks, http://gil.ipswichcity.gld.gov.au/
3 'The New Human Condition', *New Scientist* supplement 15 Oct 1994.
4 Keys, Sir William 1995, *A Flower In Winter*, Allen and Unwin, Sydney.
5 Draft Summary of Internet and Internet Related Projects 1995, Commonwealth Internet Reference Group, Feb.
6 Department of Social Security, *Community Information Network*, Canberra.
7 Office of Government Information and Advertising 1995, *Guidelines for Australian Government Information Activities*, Feb, Canberra.
8 Australian Urban and Regional Development Review 1994, *New Homes for Old*, Strategy Paper #1, Commonwealth of Australia.
9 Storey, J. 1995, *Designing for Durability—in Pursuit of Sustainability.* Paper given at Catalyst '95—Rethinking the Built Environment, conference organised by the Faculty of Environmental Design, University of Canberra.
10 IIR Conference 1995, 'Formulating a market strategy to capture the over 50s consumer', 27 Sept, Sydney.
11 Gibson, D. 1995, 'User Rights and the Frail Aged. *Journal of Applied Philosophy*, 12(1): 1–11.
12 Day, A. and Day, L. 1994, *The Lay of the Land' Older Age Structures, Environment and Social Change: Opportunities for Australia and the Netherlands in the 21st Century,* NIDI Hofstee Lecture Series 2, June, Amsterdam.

Further reading

As well as the references indicated at the end of each chapter, we provide a list of other readings to which readers may wish to refer. There is a concentration on Australian sources with just an indication of the resources available in the international literature. The list is eclectic and readers may well wish to search any good library list around key words like 'age' and 'ageing' to develop their own list.

Journals

The only specialist Australian journal is the *Australian Journal on Ageing* published by the Council of the Ageing, 2/3 Bowen Cres., Melbourne Vic 3004.

Other generalist medical and social science journals are increasingly publishing papers on ageing as indicated by references in this book.

Other regular and special publications

Regular publications and special series of the Australian Bureau of Statistics and the Australian Institute of Health and Welfare are important sources of new data and facts on ageing, in particular:

Australia's Health 1996. The fifth biennial health report of the Australian Institute of Health and Welfare, AGPS, Canberra.

Australia's Welfare & Services Assistance 1995. The second biennial health report of the Australian Institute of Health and Welfare, AGPS, Canberra.

Mathers, Colin assisted by de Looper, Michael (1994) *Health differentials among older Australians*, AGPS, Canberra.

Zhibin Liu, (1996) *Length of stay in Australian nursing homes*, Australian Institute of Health and Welfare, Canberra.

Recent Australian books include:

Kendig, Hal and McCallum, John (eds) (1990) *Grey policy: Australian policies for an ageing society*, Allen & Unwin, Sydney.

Minichiello, Victor, Alexander, Loris, Jones, Deirdre (eds) (1992) *Gerontology: A multidisciplinary approach*, Prentice-Hall of Australia, Sydney.

Rowlands, Donald T. (1991) *Ageing in Australia*, Longman Cheshire, Australia.

Sax, Sidney, (1993) *Ageing and public policy in Australia*, Allen & Unwin, Sydney.

Techuva, Karen, Stanislavsky, Yury, Kendig, Hal (1994) *Towards healthy aging: Literature review*, Collins Dove, Blackburn.

New books continually appear so readers should check library lists and reviews in journals.

International books include:

Binstock, Robert H., George, Linda, L. (1990) *Handbook of ageing and social sciences*, (3rd edn), Academic Press, SanDiego, Ca.

Callahan, Daniel, (1987) *Setting Limits: Medical goals in an ageing society*, Simon & Schuster Inc, New York.

Challis, David, Davies, Bleddyn, Traske, Karen (1994) *Community care: New agendas and challenges from the UK and overseas*, Arena, Aldershot, Hants.

Day, Alice T. (1991) *Remarkable survivors: Insights into successful ageing among women*, Urban Institute Press, Washington, DC.

Eekelaar, John and Pearl, David (1989) *An Ageing World: Dilemmas and challenges for law and social policy*, Clarendon Press: Oxford.

Friedan, Betty (1993) *The fountain of age*, Simon and Schuster, New York.

Laslett, Peter (1989) *A Fresh Map of Life: The emergence of the third age*, Weidenfield and Nicolson, London.

Netton, Ann and Beecham, Jennifer (1993) *Costing Community Care: Theory and Practice*, Gower, Aldershot.

Organisation for Economic Cooperation and Development (1994) *Caring for frail elderly people: New directions in care*, Organisation for Economic Cooperation and Development, Paris.

Schulz, James, H. (1992) *The economics of ageing*, (5th edn), Auburn House, Westport, Conn.

Tilak, Shrinivas (1989) *Religion and Ageing in the Indian Tradition*, State University of New York, Albany, New York.

Winslow, Gerald R., Walters, James W. (1993) *Facing limits: Ethics and health care for the elderly*, Westview Press, Boulder, Col.

New Doctoral and to a lesser extent Masters theses should be considered, for example:

Nay, Rhonda (1993) *Benevolent oppression: Lived experiences of nursing home life*, University of New South Wales, School of Sociology.

Commonwealth Government publications

The weight of Australian publications from the Commonwealth Government have driven the new policy agenda on ageing for the last 10 or more years. Scoping and evaluation studies have been important initiatives in reforms. Some limited examples show the diversity of materials available.

Aged care reform strategy mid-term review 1990–91: Report, Commonwealth Department of Health, Housing and Community Services, AGPS, Canberra, 1991.

Ageing research directory 1990, Office for the Aged, Department of Community Services and Health, AGPS, Canberra, 1990

Australian ageing research directory 1993, Office for the Aged, Department of Health, Housing, Local Government and Community Services, 4th edn, AGPS, Canberra 1993. (Note: A new directory is in preparation in 1996.)

Care choices for older Australians: A guide to services provided by the Commonwealth Department of Health, Housing and Community Services, Australia. Department of Health, Housing and Community Services, AGPS, Canberra, 1994.

Focus on families: Caring in families—support for persons who are older or have disabilities, Australian Bureau of Statistics, Canberra, 1995.

It's my place: Older people talk about their homes, by Barbara Davison et al., AGPS, Canberra, 1993.

Medication for the older person, report of the Health Care Committee Expert Panel for Health Care of the Elderly, National Health and Medical Research Council (Australia), Canberra, 1994.

Report: Working Party on the Protection of Frail Older People in the Community, AGPS, Canberra, 1994.

Resident classification instrument documentation consultation, Macri, Sue & Thompson Health Care Pty Ltd, Australia, Department of Health, Housing, Local Government and Community Services.

Review of the structure of nursing home funding arrangements: Stage 1, Bob Gregory, AGPS, Canberra, 1993.

The balance of care: A framework for planning, Mid-Term Review of Aged Care Reform Strategy 1990–91, Australia, Department of Community Services and Health, Canberra, 1991.

The problem of dementia in Australia, prepared by A.F. Jorm and A.S. Henders, 3rd edn, AGPS, Canberra, 1993.

Towards a national agenda for carers: Report on the workshop (AGAC), Department of Human Services and Health, Aged and Community Care Division and Office of Disability 1996, AGPS, Canberra.

Who can decide? Legal decision making for others (AGAC), Robin Creyke, AGPS, Canberra, 1995.

There are also important publications from state governments and other bodies which need to be considered. There are, in short, a wealth of materials on ageing which can be accessed effectively through any good library.

Index

Printed and bound by CPI Group (UK) Ltd, Croydon, CR0 4YY

23/10/2024

01777665-0006